Evidence Based Health Care Workbook: understanding research

For individual and group learning

Based on the book *How to Read a Paper*

Trisha Greenhalgh and Anna Donald

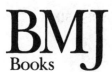

BMJ
Books

First published in 2000
Second impression 2000
Third impression 2002
by the BMJ Publishing Group, BMA House, Tavistock Square,
London WC1H 9JR

www.bmjbooks.com

British Library Cataloguing in Publication Data

A catalogue record for this book is available from the
British Library

ISBN: 0-7279-1447-2

All *BMJ* articles are reproduced by permission of the *BMJ*

All articles from *Evidence Based Medicine* are reproduced by permission of BMJ/ACP-ASIM

Typeset by Phoenix Photosetting, Chatham, Kent
Printed and bound by J. W. Arrowsmith Ltd, Bristol

Evidence Based Health Care Workbook: understanding research

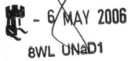
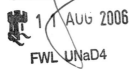
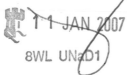
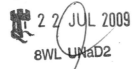
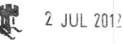

Contents

Preface   vii
Acknowledgements   viii

Unit 1: *Using this book in learning and teaching*   1
Unit 2: *The principles and practice of evidence based health care*   11
Unit 3: *Approaching the literature*   37
Unit 4: *Papers that report drug trials (randomised controlled trials of therapy)* 59
Unit 5: *Numbers needed to treat, odds ratios, and confidence intervals*   79
Unit 6: *Papers that address prognosis or harm (cohort studies)*   89
Unit 7: *Papers that report diagnostic or screening tests*   97
Unit 8: *Papers that summarise other papers (systematic review and meta-analysis)* 111
Unit 9: *Papers that go beyond numbers (qualitative research)*   131
Unit 10: *Papers that analyse very rare events (case control studies)*   145

Notes for tutors   153
Model answers for checklists   157
Index   163

Contents

Preface

This workbook has developed from the course material prepared for the London Workshops on Teaching Evidence Based Health Care. These very popular workshops have been running since February 1996 and are based on a model originally developed at McMaster University in the early 1990s. Their scope and format are described further in the reprint "Workshops for teaching evidence based practice" (page 8).

No workbook can be all things to all individuals or all groups and a book that claims to offer all the "answers" in such a rapidly changing field as evidence based health care would quickly become out of date. Our aim in preparing this workbook was to provide a resource for individual reflection and group discussion, based mainly on a wide selection of classic and/or controversial papers previously published in the *British Medical Journal* and elsewhere.

We hope that the open-ended nature of the study units, the lists of further reading, and the range of suggestions for how to use the material in interactive group work, will allow students and tutors to explore new ways of teaching and learning.

Note that we have deliberately not tried to incorporate into this workbook a textbook of evidence based health care. We believe that an understanding of conceptually complex topics must be *built* through reflection, discussion and synthesis rather than *consumed* in ready-made bites. There will be many times when you wish to pursue the theoretical aspects of clinical epidemiology in more detail. For this, we recommend one of the many articles, chapters, and textbooks listed at the end of each unit. Our own work includes Trisha's *How to read a paper: the basics of evidence based medicine* and our joint publication *A hands-on guide to evidence based health care: practice and implementation.*

We would welcome your suggestions on how to improve this book. Please write to us c/o the publishers or email us on ebp@ucl.ac.uk.

Trisha Greenhalgh
Anna Donald

Acknowledgements

This workbook would not have been published without the input of many friends, supporters, and professional colleagues. We hope we have remembered to list everyone below and apologise in advance to anyone we have inadvertently omitted.

At the time of writing, the first four London Workshops on Teaching Evidence Based Health Care (organised by Trisha Greenhalgh) had offered training in evidence based health care to 400 delegates and 90 small group tutors from a total of 17 countries and 15 different professional disciplines including medicine, nursing, management, informatics, pharmacy, osteopathy, philosophy, and mathematics. We are planning to welcome a further 120 delegates to the 5th London Workshop in March 2000.

We are grateful to the many delegates and tutors on these workshops and other courses, too numerous to mention individually, who have given us detailed feedback on what works (and what doesn't) when trying to learn (and learning how to teach) the principles of evidence based practice in a multidisciplinary setting. We acknowledge the enthusiasm and hard work of Professor David Sackett, who brought the original idea for the workshops from Canada, helped us train our first group of tutors, and offered invaluable support during our first workshop in early 1996. We are also indebted to the members of the evidence based health email discussion list for numerous ideas for "good teaching material" freely shared and discussed.

Professor Lewis Elton taught us a lot about how students learn. He also, by his inspirational example, taught us how to teach (and how to lecture). Marcia Rigby has organised the London workshops since 1997 and provided tireless administrative support for this and other publications.

Mary Banks and her team from BMJ Books tolerated our idiosyncracies, rushed the manuscript to the printers in record time, and did a lot more besides. Our families supported us throughout.

UNIT 1 — *Using this book in learning and teaching*

BEFORE YOU START – DEFINE YOUR AIMS AND OBJECTIVES

It ought to be self-evident that any formal educational experience – meeting, seminar, course, conference, lecture, learning set, journal club or whatever – should have clearly defined aims, i.e. broad goals for what the organisers hope to achieve. In addition, each individual session should have explicit learning objectives (i.e. specific things that the learners should *know* or be able to *do* by the end of that session).

If you are organising an educational meeting and you are unable to commit yourself in writing to precisely what participants should expect to get out of it, you should not be surprised if they express confusion and dissatisfaction! If you are studying alone, you will almost certainly find that defining your overall aim and setting particular objectives for each study session will make your learning more effective and enjoyable.

As the authors of this workbook, it is not our place to define in any detail your own aims or objectives (or those of the group you intend to teach). We encourage you to think carefully about the aims of your course as a whole and about the specific learning objectives for each session.

AIMS

Here are some examples of aims for which this workbook might provide one resource.

Sample aims for a one-week short course on teaching evidence based health care (EBHC)

- To provide an environment where participants from a range of backgrounds can explore different educational models for teaching evidence based practice and discuss the design, development, and maintenance of appropriate curricula.
- To allow participants to develop their own skills in question framing, critical appraisal, database searching, and teaching as part of a lifelong professional development process.
- To encourage long-term networking and resource sharing between individuals and institutions whose common aim is the effective teaching of evidence based practice.

Sample aims for a learning set that meets for a half-day session on a regular basis to develop a programme of clinical governance in a health service organisation

- To provide regular protected time and a safe environment in which participants can explore the principles of evidence based health care and apply these to their own working practice.
- To allow participants to develop relevant skills in question framing, critical appraisal, and database searching and apply these skills to real clinical problems.

- To build an efficient, multidisciplinary, task-oriented team that is able to identify and draw upon the knowledge and skills of individual members in developing and implementing evidence based clinical policy within the organisation.

Sample aims for an individual who wishes to improve their own skills in evidence based health care

- To become familiar with the theoretical principles of evidence based health care and the main controversies surrounding its application in practice, in order to make an informed decision on how I should use research evidence in my unit or organisation.
- To pass an undergraduate or postgraduate examination or gain a particular vocational qualification.
- To improve my own practice in a particular clinical area or to develop an evidence based clinical guideline or policy for myself and my team.

LEARNING OBJECTIVES

You will find suggestions for learning objectives listed at the beginning of each unit. An example of a learning objective is

"By the end of this study unit on critical appraisal of research evidence [which involves reading and evaluating a paper describing an original research trial], we hope you will be able to state the purpose of the trial, describe the methods used by the investigators and comment on their validity, identify the main sources of bias and confounding, and estimate the magnitude and precision of the results."

Because learning objectives refer to what the learner should be able to do, they should be expressed as a set of verbs (such as "state", "describe", "comment", "identify", and so on). If you plan to measure the extent to which the objectives have been achieved (for example, by means of a formal test, examination or summative assessment), the learning objectives should be defined in terms of measurable tasks that have a reasonably clear threshold for demonstrating competence (i.e. the learner can be readily classified as either able or unable to perform the task). The objective "understand Bayes' theorem" is much less helpful, for example, than "demonstrate how Bayes' theorem can inform the judicious use of diagnostic tests in the clinical encounter".

SET ARTICLES

1. Bligh J. Problem-based, small group learning. *BMJ* 1995; **311**: 342–3.
2. Greenhalgh T. Workshops for teaching evidence based practice. *Evidence Based Med* 1997; **2**: 7–8.

LEARNING IN A GROUP

The reprint on pages 6–7 offers a number of reasons why we are enthusiastic about group work for learning and teaching evidence based health care. Educationists talk about "superficial learning" (characterised by the ability to recognise, recall, and reproduce facts) and "deep learning" (characterised by the ability to perform more complex tasks such as analysis, synthesis, reflection, comparison, and application of knowledge gained in one context to an entirely new context).

Group work is a particularly effective method for supporting deep learning because it encourages (indeed, requires) the activities of listening, questioning, explaining, comparing, consolidating, summarising, and evaluating.

The detailed theoretical principles of small group work are beyond the scope of this book but we suggest that both tutors and group members should be familiar with the basics before starting out on an intensive learning experience.

Remember

- Small group work should be *fun*.
- Small group work is usually *exhausting*.
- Small group work can be *effective*.

To make it more fun, less exhausting, and more effective, we suggest five tips.

1. Get to know each other.
   - What are our names, professional backgrounds, and interests?
   - What relevant skills, experience or perspectives do individual members have?
   - What were our individual objectives in coming on the course and/or joining the group?
2. Set some ground rules.
   - When will each session start and finish? How important is it that we all turn up to every session and that we start and finish on time? How will we cope with members who turn up late or irregularly?
   - How will we run each session? Will members take it in turns to present or lead sessions? How about presenting in pairs?
   - How will we deal with interruptions and distractions (for example, "bleeps", mobile phones, people "just popping out")?
   - How will we use our designated tutor or facilitator (if we have one)? If we don't have one, should one of us take on that role?
   - What methods (formal presentations, informal discussions, role play) and technologies (flip chart, video, computer) will we use for our learning?
   - Do we have a specific task to complete (for example, a project to do) that has been set by someone outside the group and, if so, what are our terms of reference towards that individual?
3. Be aware of two aspects of the learning.
   - *Content – what* is being covered. What is the clinical topic, what dimension of the problem is the focus of discussion, what depth is it being covered in, etc?
   - *Process – how* it is being covered. Who is speaking, who is listening (and who isn't), are any points of view being unreasonably dismissed, is the speaker simply stating their opinion or offering reasoned argument, etc?
   You may wish to delineate a means of commenting on process that is distinct from routine input on content. The McMaster group developed the expressions "Time out" and "Time in" for this. For example, the tutor might say, "Time out. Henry and Fred, the points you are making are very good, but you seem to be having your own dialogue rather than including the rest of the group. Time in."
4. Have a broad structure in mind for every session.
   - Set the agenda for the session (leaving time for practical things such as shifting furniture, moving to break-out rooms, and refreshments, as well as the other tasks listed below).
   - Agree on the topic to be covered, the methods to be used, the roles of the group members and tutor, and the learning objectives (see page 2).
   - Run the session, modifying the objectives as you go along if necessary (for example, if it emerges that they were unrealistic). Use the Time out / Time in markers if you find them useful.

- Evaluate this session.
- Plan the next session.
5. Establish and follow rules for giving feedback to a group member.
    - Timing
        - Allocate protected time during or after the session for feedback.
        - Try to give feedback as soon after the event as possible.
    - Packaging. When giving negative feedback:
        - Use the "criticism sandwich": begin and end your feedback on a positive note (for example, "It was a good idea to try a role play here. Unfortunately I felt my brief was ambiguous, and I think quite a few others felt the same. As a result I felt the session didn't hang together. But still, we all got to know each other better and we've learnt some lessons for next time").
        - Use "I" and give your experience of the behaviour (for example, "When you said ..., I felt that you were ...").
    - Content
        - Stick to one or two points.
        - Confine your comments to things that can be changed. There is no point saying "You've got an awful sense of humour", but you could say, "I felt it was inappropriate to make a joke at that point in your presentation".
        - Describe specific behaviours and give examples ("You stood up and spoke loudly") rather than assigning motives ("You were trying to intimidate her").
        - Suggest alternative behaviours ("Perhaps you could have asked everyone at that point if they were still with you").
    - Self-awareness
        - Remember that feedback says a lot about you as well as about the person to whom it is directed.
        - Ask yourself, "Why am I giving this feedback?". If you want to show how much you know or contribute generally to the topic under discussion, the feedback session is not the place to do it.

LEARNING ON YOUR OWN

Although this book was originally developed as a resource for small group work, there is no reason why you should not use it for individual study. Some people can study very effectively on their own; others find they need more interaction with fellow students. Research papers and review articles can be very dry and uninspiring. Arguments and discussions about what particular texts mean, as well as stories about real-life practice ("When we tried that ..."), are all ways of engaging with the text and consolidating the learning.

If you are following a self-directed course of study and do not have the benefit of regular contact with a tutor or fellow students, the following tips may help you achieve deeper understanding of the material presented here.

We strongly advise you to use this workbook alongside a general textbook of clinical epidemiology or evidence based practice such as the selection listed below.

Set aside regular protected time for your studies. If you are working for an examination, draw up a timetable that allows you to cover all the main topics. If you fail to cover one topic to your satisfaction, decide whether to abandon it or give it more time by compromising another topic. As described on page 2, make sure you define specific objectives for your learning.

When you read an article, make notes on its main message and list the points you do not understand. You may, at this point, need to look things up in reference textbooks or approach an expert in the subject. (Keep a running list of questions so you do not have to disturb your expert too many times!).

When you have finished reading an article, think about how you might apply its message in practice. How would you explain its message to a group of students who are new to the topic? How would you persuade a colleague to change their practice in the light of the results? What might be the argument of a colleague who was resistant to change and how would you respond? If you were of the opinion that "evidence based medicine is a load of rubbish", what would your reaction to this article be?

By going through mental exercises like this, you are creating, in effect, an imaginary group of people with different perspectives, opinions, and knowledge levels about the subject and by constructing an imaginary response to them, you will achieve a deeper understanding of the topic.

FURTHER READING

Books on EBHC

Donald A, Greenhalgh T. *A hands-on guide to evidence based health care: practice and implementation.* Oxford: Blackwell, 1999.
(*A textbook designed for the busy clinician or manager, with major sections on the practicalities of achieving EBHC in the real world.*)

Greenhalgh T. *How to read a paper: the basics of evidence based medicine.* London: BMJ Books, 1997.
(*An introductory text designed for those with no previous background in EBHC, intended for both medical and non-medical readers.*)

Sackett DL, Haynes RB, Guyatt GH, Tugwell P. *Clinical epidemiology: a basic science for clinical medicine.* London: Little, Brown, 1991.
(*A comprehensive reference text covering detailed aspects of EBHC and including an extensive section on professional development, designed primarily for doctors.*)

Sackett DL, Richardson WS, Rosenberg WMC, Haynes RB. *Evidence-based medicine: how to practise and teach EBM.* London: Churchill Livingstone, 1997.
(*A pocket-sized summary text of the principles of EBM, containing tips for teaching.*)

Books and articles on teaching and group work

Crosby J. Learning in small groups. Association for Medical Education in Europe Education Guide No. 8. *Medical Teacher* 1999; **19**: 189–202.
Elwyn G, Greenhalgh T, Macfarlane F, Koppel S. *Groups: a hands-on guide to small group work in education, management, and research.* Oxford: Radcliffe, 1999 (in press).
Eraut M. *Developing professional knowledge and competence.* London: Falmer Press, 1993.

Problem based, small group learning

An idea whose time has come

Problem based learning is an educational method that uses problems as the starting point for student learning.[1] In medical education these problems are usually clinical and integrate basic science with clinical thinking. Such methods have been used since the 1960s, when the medical school at McMaster, Ontario, first introduced an entirely new approach to medical education.[2]

Identifying material for a course of problem based learning requires teachers to analyse their discipline for the critical elements that are essential to medical practice. Once such core elements have been identified, clinical problems can be composed and supporting learning activities (such as lectures, practicals, workshops, and clinical attachments) arranged. Students learn by seeking solutions to the problems. To do this they work in small groups to break the problem into its constituent parts, identifying relations and connections along the way. Individual learning and attendance at timetabled activities follow, with students searching for answers to questions they have raised themselves during the analysis. Validation of learning takes place in the small group under the eye of the tutor.

Problem based learning has spread to continental Europe, the Middle and Far East, and Australia[3] but has not taken root in the United Kingdom. Newly established medical schools are most likely to use problem based learning, although complete conversion within a traditional curriculum and within existing resources is possible.[4] A "dual track" approach has been successfully used in several schools (for example, the University of New Mexico).[5] Evidence of its effectiveness in producing medical graduates comparable to those produced by traditional programmes has been sporadically produced, and concerns have yet to be assuaged that it fails to influence the development of general problem solving skills. A recurring concern about problem based learning is that it costs more in terms of staff time; however, its effect is not to increase teaching time but rather to change how this time is spent — for example, teachers using problem based learning spend up to 40% more time working with students.[6] Assessment is another concern. The experience at McMaster, where feedback on progress is prominent, shows that knowledge remains an essential foundation for learning and that it must be tested without styles of student learning being unwittingly distorted.[7]

With publication of the results of Harvard Medical School's evaluation of its new pathway programme[8] and two recent major review papers, we are still no clearer about the effects of the method on problem solving skills. Harvard used multiple measures, including questionnaires, interviews, and videotapes of consultations, to compare students on the two year preclinical component of the new pathway with their peers randomly allocated to the traditional programme. They found that the students allocated to the new pathway reflected more on their learning, memorised less than their peers, and preferred active learning. Interpersonal skills, psychosocial knowledge, and attitudes towards patients (for example, patient centredness and empathy) were better in the new pathway group, and the students felt more stimulated, challenged, and satisfied. There were no differences, in terms of biomedical knowledge, between the two groups of students in performance in the National Board of Medical Examiners' part I examination. New pathway students reported less cramming of knowledge before exams; better retention in the months afterwards; and, because the result

of the exams was a pass or fail rather than a grade, feeling less threatened.[9,10]

Promoting enjoyable learning

Although the authors recognised that students adapt to the learning environment in which they find themselves, the new pathway students reported significantly greater autonomy, more innovation and involvement, and similar work pressures to those reported by matched controls after two years. The new pathway students were also more sure of themselves in handling uncertainty. Students on the traditional curriculum were more likely to use the key words "non-relevant, passive, and boring" to describe their preclinical experience. New pathway students, however, reported that some interpersonal aspects of tutorial work caused frustration and anxiety, as did concerns over what and how much to study.

Other findings echo these from Harvard. Two recent review papers, one examining over 100 papers about problem based learning and the other reporting on its psychological basis, have offered medical teachers a broad reference base from which to draw conclusions. For Albanese and Mitchell, concerns about the costs of implementation and about the cognitive processes that some students may develop balance evidence of adequate learning of basic science and the development of self learning skills.[11] They recommend caution when considering curriculum-wide conversion to problem based learning, suggesting teacher directed learning of basic science alongside the exploration of clinical cases with problem based learning.

Norman and Schmidt, from McMaster (Canada) and Maastricht (Netherlands), report that students using problem based learning have a greater intrinsic interest in learning, their self directed learning skills are enhanced (and are retained), and basic science concepts are better integrated into the solving of clinical problems.[12,13] They also report that, although the problem based learning format may initially reduce the amount that students learn, subsequent retention of knowledge is increased. The review emphasises the importance of students puzzling through problems to learn concepts and suggests that individual learning and groups without tutors may both have a role in the future.

Both reviews emphatically support the psychosocial effect that problem based learning has on students and teaching staff. The attitudes of teachers and the atmosphere of cooperation in a problem based learning curriculum mean that graduates report that they find the "learning environment more stimulating and more humane" than do graduates of conventional schools. With undergraduate medical education currently carrying a health warning because of the stress and anxiety exhibited by students and young graduates, any educational process that promotes enjoyment of learning without loss of basic knowledge and skills must be a good thing.[14-16]

The General Medical Council has strongly recommended reform of the curriculum in Britain.[17] It wants substantially less teaching of factual information. Instead, it wants an integrated "core" curriculum based on body systems, with active learning driven by curiosity and a greater use of the critical evaluation of evidence. Special study modules will augment core and offer students in depth opportunities to study scientific method and research.

British medical schools are thus under pressure, not only to reform their curriculum but also to change the process of

Originally published in *BMJ* 1995; **311**: 342–3.

learning. The response so far has been encouraging. Study guides and learning contracts are being introduced in Dundee; clinical skills units are planned or in place at St Bartholomew's Hospital and in Dundee, Leeds, and Liverpool; computer assisted learning is a feature of Aberdeen's plans; and multidisciplinary groups characterise planning for reform of the syllabus in many schools. Sheffield is piloting a structured supervision project, and special study modules have been developed in Birmingham, Edinburgh, Leicester, and Manchester. Manchester has already introduced problem oriented group work into its first year course; Glasgow and Liverpool are committed to problem based learning as a major learning strategy from 1996; and other schools are actively considering its introduction. As far as Britain is concerned, problem based learning seems at last to be coming in from the cold.

JOHN BLIGH
Professor

University Medical Education Unit,
Royal Liverpool University Hospital,
Liverpool L69 3BX

1 Barrows HS, Tamblyn RN. *Problem-based learning: an approach to medical education.* New York: Springer, 1980.
2 Neufield VR, Woodward CA, MacLeod SM. The McMaster MD programme: a case study in renewal in medical education. *Acad Med* 1989;**64**:423–32.
3 Walton HJ, Matthews MB, eds. Essentials of problem-based learning. *Med Educ* 1989;23:542–58.
4 Des Marchais JE, Bureau MA, Dumais B, Pigeon G. From traditional to problem-based learning: a case report of a complete curriculum reform. *Med Educ* 1992;**26**:190–9.
5 Kaufman A, ed. *Implementing problem-based medical education: lessons from successful innovations.* New York: Springer, 1985.
6 Mennin SP, Martinez-Burrola N. The cost of problem-based vs traditional medical education. *Med Educ* 1986;**20**:187–94.
7 Blake JM, Norman GR, Smith EKM. Report card from McMaster: student evaluation at a problem-based medical school. *Lancet* 1995;**345**:899–902.
8 Moore GT, Block SD, Style CB, Mitchell R. The influence of the new pathway curriculum on Harvard medical students. *Acad Med* 1994;**69**:983–9.
9 Tosteson DC, Adelstein SJ, Carver ST, eds. *New pathways to medical education: learning to learn at Harvard Medical School.* Cambridge: Harvard University Press, 1994.
10 McManus C. New pathways to medical education: learning to learn at Harvard Medical School [book review]. *BMJ* 1995;**311**:67.
11 Albanese MA, Mitchell S. Problem-based learning: a review of literature on its outcomes and implementation issues. *Acad Med* 1993;**68**:52–81.
12 Norman GR, Schmidt HG. The psychological basis of problem-based learning: a review of the evidence. *Acad Med* 1992;**67**:557–65.
13 Schmidt HG, Norman GR, Boshuizen HPA. A cognitive perspective on medical expertise: theory and implications. *Acad Med* 1990;**65**:611–21.
14 Weatherall DJ. The inhumanity of medicine. *BMJ* 1994;308:1671–2.
15 Wolf TM, Randall HM, von Almen K, Tynes LL. Perceived mistreatment and attitude change by graduating medical students: a retrospective study. *Med Educ* 1991;**25**:182–90.
16 Dowie R, Charlton B. *The making of a doctor.* Oxford: Oxford University Press, 1994.
17 General Medical Council. *Tomorrow's doctors. Report of the Education Committee.* London: GMC, 1993.

Workshops for teaching evidence-based practice

Evidence-based practice is based on a systematic approach to the literature with focused and answerable questions, critical appraisal of the validity and usefulness of what is found, application of the results to real patients and real at-risk populations, and evaluation of the practitioner's performance (1). This approach, which relegates content (the factual things we need to know) below process (how we go about learning and applying, the facts), requires different skills and attitudes from those that most of us had when we left university. How do people acquire these new skills and attitudes, and how can they be most effectively taught?

The basic tenets of clinical epidemiology were taught to me 15 years ago at Oxford University in a 2-week block titled "Community Medicine"; the course had the worst attendance figures in the entire undergraduate curriculum. We were issued a set of equations and potted definitions that were filed — along with the porphyrin chain and other medical megaliths — in a binder labelled "Night Before File," the contents of which would be memorised, regurgitated, and gratefully forgotten as the examination season came and went.

Much of the work done in the field of evidence-based medicine since 1980 has been aimed at getting clinical epidemiology out of the "Night Before File" and into the clinic; the operating theatre; and (most difficult of all) the everyday vocabulary of managers, commissioners, and purchasers. Practised at the bedside and around the contracting table, evidence-based medicine forces health professionals to unite a scientific (hypothetico-deductive) paradigm with one that is hermeneutic (narrative-interpretive).

Here is an extract from one of the worksheets used in the 2nd U.K. Workshop on Teaching Evidence-Based Health Care, held at University College London (UCL) Medical School in February 1996:

"Read the clinical scenario [about a patient aged 18 months with a single febrile seizure] and the attached case-control study on the long-term prognosis after febrile seizure in infants. Decide whether and to what extent a single uncomplicated febrile seizure increases the risk of subsequent epilepsy, and using a role-play or other appropriate teaching techniques, decide how you would convey this information to the child's parents."

In this and other clinical problems, practitioners of evidence-based medicine must take on aspects of the discipline that do not come naturally and for which they were not originally trained. The non-numerate must gain some grasp of statistics, whereas those who like to add up figures must learn to find the source of the figures and apply them to individual circumstances. Clinicians who make decisions on the basis of precise statistical likelihoods must, if they are to share decision making with a truly informed patient, find a way to express complex concepts in jargon-free terminology and to incorporate patient preferences into their probability trees.

Blind ideology did not prompt us at UCL to teach these multidimensional skills through the technique of problem-based, small-group, self-directed learning (2, 3). To achieve sustained behaviour change in fields outside of the practitioner's immediate area of expertise, such issues as confidence-building, teamwork, and intellectual initiative must not be treated as peripheral to the course content (4). McMaster University Medical School (5) in Canada and the Harvard New Pathway programme (6) in the United States have shown that undergraduate students taught by problem-based methods reflect more on their learning, memorise less, and report greater stimulation and satisfaction with the course than those allocated to a predominantly talk-and-chalk curriculum.

We were initially sceptical about re-placing the traditional lecture-based conference format with a largely blank timetable in which the delegates' first task was to sit down in small groups and decide 1) what they needed to know and 2) how they were going to teach it to each other. We provided each group of 8 with little more than a seminar room and a flip chart. But by day 2 of the 6-day workshop, eminent professors were happily engrossed in pretending to be medical students not understanding likelihood ratios; geriatricians were role-playing as either patients who had had a stroke or the managers charged with rehabilitating them; and a group of public health physicians were, within the safety of their group, staging a mock press conference to assuage public anxiety about the safety of measles-mumps-rubella vaccine.

The delegates, who created these diverse teaching scenarios from their own experiences, were simultaneously required to consider the artificial situation they had created ("You are medical students; I am teaching you about likelihood ratios") and the meta-situation ("I am someone who is learning to teach; how could I do this more effectively?"). Each group member had an allocated role to play in the simulated teaching scenario, but they and the tutors could at any stage call a "time-out" and comment on the meta-situation.

The first U.K. workshop to follow the McMaster University model was held at Oxford University in June 1995. It led to the formation of the U.K. Consortium on Teaching Evidence-Based Medicine (supported by an educational grant from the North Thames Regional Office) in which centres throughout the United Kingdom collaborate to share educational materials (some of which will soon be available over the Internet [e-mail to http://cebm.jr2.ox.ac.uk]), to plan workshops, and to develop methods to evaluate their success. A third workshop was held in Oxford this July, and the UCL group will host the fourth at the Royal College of

Originally published in *Evidence-Based Medicine* 1997; 2: 7–8.

Physicians in February 1997. A core textbook has been published (7), and we hope to explore the use of more imaginative teaching materials (such as video scenarios) in future workshops.

The responses to questionnaires issued before the UCL workshop showed that, for many delegates, implementation of evidence-based medicine at their home institutions was limited as much by lack of time, information technology skills, "political acceptance," and confidence as by lack of knowledge (8). Postworkshop responses showed that despite these barriers, 40% of the 88 delegates intended to introduce new teaching programmes in clinical schools, health authorities, or National Health Service trusts, and of these delegates, all but one planned to use small-group, problem-based learning in substantial portions of the curriculum.

An important challenge for medical educators in the United Kingdom is to recognise that the competent student (and clinician) is one who knows how to cope with an immense and rapidly changing body of knowledge and not one who excels in recalling the traditional or memorising the ephemeral. The deans of medical and nursing schools must develop an infrastructure that allows problem-based, self-directed learning methods to develop within the didactic, lecture-based curricula, which have seen no fundamental changes for 2 centuries or more. As one delegate asked me without a trace of irony, "Is there any way of having small-group seminars when you haven't got any seminar rooms?"

The UCL workshop achieved undeniable short-term gains in terms of the number of complex scientific articles read and understood (estimated at around 15 per delegate), new skills acquired (35% of the delegates before the workshop and 85% after were confident in using MEDLINE), altered attitudes (particularly to multidisciplinary learning), and exposure to new educational techniques. Despite these gains, the long-term influence of this type of workshop on the educational strategies used in traditional British medical schools and the behaviour of busy health professionals in the National Health Service has still to be determined.

At our 6-month reunion workshop this October, our first question to delegates will be this: Has the evidence-based medicine you learned in this workshop been incorporated into your daily practice and has its key message been passed on to others in a way that they can understand? Or have your notes, worksheets, and good intentions been placed back on the shelf next to the "Night Before File"?

For further information about the 4th U.K. Workshop on Teaching Evidence-Based Practice, contact us by e-mail at ebp@ucl.ac.uk.

Trisha Greenhalgh, MD

References
1. Sackett DL, Haynes RB. Evidence-Based Medicine. 1995 Nov-Dec; 1:5–6.
2. Bligh J. BMJ. 1995;311:342–3.
3. Vernon DT, Blake RL. Acad Med. 1993;68:550–63.
4. Norman GR, Schmidt HG. Acad Med. 1992;67:557–65.
5. Donald A, ed. Evidence-based medicine: a report from McMaster University Medical School and Teaching Hospitals: becoming better, faster, happier docs. Oxford: Anglia and Oxford; 1994.
6. Tosteson DC, Adelstein SJ, Carver ST, eds. New pathways to medical education: learning to learn at Harvard Medical School. Cambridge, Massachusetts: Harvard University Press; 1994.
7. Sackett DL, Richardson WS, Rosenberg WM, Haynes RB. Evidence-based medicine: how to practice and teach EBM. London: Churchill-Livingstone; 1997.
8. 2nd U.K. Workshop on Teaching Evidence-Based Health Care: report of the workshop. Available on disc (Word for Windows format) from the Department of Primary Health Care, University College London Medical School, Whittington Hospital, London N19 5NF England, UK. Price £7.50.

UNIT 2   *The principles and practice of evidence based health care*

SUGGESTED AIM FOR THIS SESSION

To explore different definitions of evidence based health care (EBHC) from the perspective of different professional and lay groups and to share different viewpoints on how the principles of EBHC can be applied in practice.

SUGGESTED LEARNING OBJECTIVES FOR THIS SESSION

By the end of this session, participants will be able to:
- discuss the potential strengths and weaknesses of the standard definition of EBHC as "the conscientious, judicious and explicit use of current best evidence in the care of individual patients";
- acknowledge the range of different perspectives on the nature and scope of the "evidence based" approach to clinical practice;
- analyse particular clinical scenarios from both an individual and a population perspective, in terms of the application of research-based evidence.

SET ARTICLES

1. Sackett DL, Rosenberg WC, Gray JAM, Haynes RB, Richardson WS. Evidence based medicine: what it is and what it isn't. *BMJ* 1996; **312**: 71–2.
2. Rosenberg W, Donald A. Evidence based medicine: an approach to clinical problem-solving. *BMJ* 1995; **310**: 1122–6.
3. Greenhalgh T. Is my practice evidence-based? *BMJ* 1996; **313**: 957–8.
4. Knottnerus JA, Dinant GJ. Medicine based evidence, a prerequisite for evidence based medicine. *BMJ* 1997; **315**: 1109–10.
5. Greenhalgh T. Narrative based medicine in an evidence based world. *BMJ* 1999; **318**: 323–5. [A longer version of this article is in: Greenhalgh T, Hurwitz B, eds. *Narrative based medicine: dialogue and discourse in clinical practice.* London: BMJ Books, 1998; 247–65.]

SUGGESTIONS FOR GROUP EXERCISES

1. Work initially in pairs and discuss:
   - why you decided to come on a course or workshop about EBHC;
   - what individual reservations you each have about the topic;
   - what additional information (if any) you would like about EBHC before deciding whether or not to explore the subject further or begin trying to apply it in practice.

When you have discussed in pairs, return to the group as a whole and share on a flip chart the main issues you raised in your pairs. What were the common themes? If any individual or pair holds a different viewpoint from the majority, to what extent does that reflect their different professional backgrounds, personal experiences or cultures?

2. If you have time to prepare a debate, try one of the following titles:
   - "This house believes that EBHC is just another passing fad"
   - "This house believes that EBHC is a thinly veiled exercise in rationing"
   - "This house believes that the EBHC movement owes more to evangelism than science"
3. Try a role play exercise in which those who identify strongly with particular views on EBHC take on the roles of individuals with very different views. (This is potentially a tough and emotionally difficult exercise so make sure you know and trust each other well enough to take it on. We recommend that you try it towards the end of a course rather than right at the beginning!)

SUGGESTIONS FOR INDIVIDUAL STUDY

1. Look through the range of reading material presented here. As you do so, make some rough notes about each of the pieces. Make two columns on a blank sheet of paper – one labelled "facts" and the other "values". What (if any) underlying assumptions are each of the authors making?
2. Choose one of the articles reproduced here and write a draft letter to the Editor of the *BMJ* which begins, "I would like to point out three counter-arguments...".
3. Think of a particular clinical example in your own practice (or, if you are not a clinician, an example of a health care experience you have had as a patient or carer). To what extent is the "rhetoric of EBHC" relevant (or irrelevant) to this case? How might a systematic application of best research evidence have changed the outcome and what difference would it have made to the patient?

FURTHER READING

Anon. Evidence-based medicine, in its place. *Lancet* 1995; **346**: 785.

Batstone G, Edwards M. Professional roles in promoting evidence-based practice. *Br J H Care Manag* 1996; **2**: 144–7.

Black D. The limitations to evidence. *J R Coll Physicians Lond* 1998; **32**: 23–6.

Bradley F, Field J. Evidence-based medicine. *Lancet* 1995; **346**: 838–9.

Davidoff F, Case K, Fried PW. Evidence-based medicine: why all the fuss? *Ann Intern Med* 1995; **122**: 727.

Drummond M. Evidence-based medicine and cost-effectiveness: uneasy bedfellows? *Evidence Based Med* 1998; **3**: 133.

Fahey T, Griffiths S, Peters TJ. Evidence based purchasing: understanding results of clinical trials and systematic reviews. *BMJ* 1995; **311**: 1056–9.

Feinstein AR, Horwitz R. Problems in the "evidence" of "evidence-based medicine". *Am J Med* 1998; **103**: 529–35.

Greenhalgh T. *How to read a paper: the basics of evidence-based medicine.* London: BMJ Books, 1997. See in particular Chapter 1: Why read papers at all? pages 1–12.

Hope A. Evidence based medicine and ethics. *J Med Ethics* 1995; **21**: 259–60.

Jones GW, Sagar SM. Evidence based medicine. No guidance is provided for situations for which evidence is lacking. *BMJ* 1995; **311**: 258.

McColl A, Roderick P, Gabbay J, Smith H, Moore M. Performance indicators for primary care groups: an evidence based approach. *BMJ* 1998; **317**: 1354.

Milne R, Hicks N. Evidence-based purchasing. *Evidence Based Med* 1996; **1**: 101–2.

Naylor CD. Grey zones of clinical practice: some limits to evidence-based medicine. *Lancet* 1995; **345**: 840–2.

Oxman AD, Sackett DL, Guyatt GH. Users' guides to the medical literature. I. How to get started. *JAMA* 1993; **270**: 2093–5.

Smith BH. Evidence based medicine. Quality cannot always be quantified. *BMJ* 1995; **311**: 258.

Stradling JR, Davies RJO. The unacceptable face of evidence-based medicine. *J Evaluation Clin Pract* 1997; **3**: 99–103.

Sullivan FM, MacNaughton RJ. Evidence in consultations: interpreted and individualised. *Lancet* 1996; **348**: 941–3.

Evidence based medicine: what it is and what it isn't

It's about integrating individual clinical expertise and the best external evidence

Evidence based medicine, whose philosophical origins extend back to mid-19th century Paris and earlier, remains a hot topic for clinicians, public health practitioners, purchasers, planners,and the public. There are now frequent workshops in how to practice and teach it; undergraduate[1] and postgraduate[2] training programmes are incorporating it[3] (or pondering how to do so); British centres for evidence based practice have been established or planned in adult medicine, child health, surgery, pathology, pharmacotherapy, nursing, general practice, and dentistry; the Cochrane Collaboration and Britain's Centre for Review and Dissemination in York are providing systematic reviews of the effects of health care; new evidence based practice journals are being launched; and it has become a common topic in the lay media. But enthusiasm has been mixed with some negative reaction.[4][5][6] Criticism has ranged from evidence based medicine being old hat to it being a dangerous innovation, perpetrated by the arrogant to serve cost cutters and suppress clinical freedom. As evidence based medicine continues to evolve and adapt, now is a useful time to refine the discussion of what it is and what it is not.

Evidence based medicine is the conscientious, explicit, and judicious use of current best evidence in making decisions about the care of individual patients. The practice of evidence based medicine means integrating individual clinical expertise with the best available external clinical evidence from systematic research. By individual clinical expertise we mean the proficiency and judgment that individual clinicians acquire through clinical experience and clinical practice. Increased expertise is reflected in many ways, but especially in more effective and efficient diagnosis and in the more thoughtful identification and compassionate use of individual patients' predicaments, rights, and preferences in making clinical decisions about their care. By best available external clinical evidence we mean clinically relevant research, often from the basic sciences of medicine, but especially from patient centred clinical research into the accuracy and precision of diagnostic tests (including the clinical examination), the power of prognostic markers, and the efficacy and safety of the rapeutic,rehabilitative, and preventive regimens. External clinical evidence both invalidates previously accepted diagnostic tests and treatments and replaces them with new ones that are more powerful, more accurate, more efficacious, and safer.

Good doctors use both individual clinical expertise and the best available external evidence, andneither alone is enough. Without clinical expertise, practice risks becoming tyrannised by evidence,for even excellent external evidence may be inapplicable to or inappropriate for an individual patient. .

Without current best evidence, practice risks becoming rapidly out of date, to the detriment of patients.

This description of what evidence based medicine is helps clarify what evidence based medicine is not. Evidence based medicine is neither old hat nor impossible to practice. The argument that "everyone already is doing it" falls before evidence of striking variations in both the integration of patient values into our clinical behaviour[7] and in the rates with which clinicians provide interventions

Originally published in *BMJ* 1996; **312** (7023): 71.

to their patients.[8] The difficulties that clinicians face in keeping abreast of all the medical advances reported in primary journals are obvious from a comparison of the time required for reading (for general medicine, enough to examine 19 articles per day, 365 days per year[9]) with the time available (well under an hour a week by British medical consultants, even on self reports[10]).

The argument that evidence based medicine can be conducted only from ivory towers and armchairs is refuted by audits from the front lines of clinical care where at least some inpatient clinical teams in general medicine,[11] psychiatry (J R Geddes et al, Royal College of Psychiatrists winter meeting, January 1996), and surgery (P McCulloch, personal communication) have provided evidence based care to the vast majority of their patients. Such studies show that busy clinicians who devote their scarce reading time to selective, efficient, patient driven searching, appraisal, and incorporation of the best available evidence can practice evidence based medicine.

Evidence based medicine is not "cookbook" medicine. Because it requires a bottom up approach that integrates the best external evidence with individual clinical expertise and patients' choice, it cannot result in slavish, cookbook approaches to individual patient care. External clinical evidence can inform, but can never replace, individual clinical expertise, and it is this expertise that decides whether the external evidence applies to the individual patient at all and, if so, how it should be integrated into a clinical decision. Similarly, any external guideline must be integrated with individual clinical expertise in deciding whether and how it matches the patient's clinical state, predicament, and preferences, and thus whether it should be applied. Clinicians who fear top down cookbooks will find the advocates of evidence based medicine joining them at the barricades.

Some fear that evidence based medicine will be hijacked by purchasers and managers to cut the costs of health care. This would not only be a misuse of evidence based medicine but suggests a fundamental misunderstanding of its financial consequences. Doctors practising evidence based medicine will identify and apply the most efficacious interventions to maximise the quality and quantity of life for individual patients; this may raise rather than lower the cost of their care.

Evidence based medicine is not restricted to randomised trials and meta-analyses. It involves tracking down the best external evidence with which to answer our clinical questions. To find out about the accuracy of a diagnostic test, we need to find proper cross sectional studies of patients clinically suspected of harbouring the relevant disorder, not a randomised trial. For a question about prognosis, we need proper follow up studies of patients assembled at a uniform, early point in the clinical course of their disease. And sometimes the evidence we need will come from the basic sciences such as genetics or immunology. It is when asking questions about therapy that we should try to avoid the non-experimental approaches, since these routinely lead to false positive conclusions about efficacy. Because the randomised trial, and especially the systematic review of several randomised trials, is so much more likely to inform us and so much less likely to mislead us, it has become the "gold standard" for judging whether a treatment does more good than harm. However, some questions about therapy do not require randomised trials (successful interventions for otherwise fatal conditions) or cannot wait for the trials to be conducted. And if no randomised trial has been carried out for our patient's predicament, we must follow the trail to the next best external evidence and work from there.

Despite its ancient origins, evidence based medicine remains a relatively young discipline whose positive impacts are just beginning to be validated,[12][13] and it will continue to evolve. This evolution will be enhanced as several undergraduate, postgraduate, and continuing medical education programmes adopt and adapt it to their learners' needs. These programmes, and their evaluation, will provide further information and understanding about what evidence based medicine is and is not.

Professor, NHS Research and Development Centre for Evidence Based Medicine, Oxford Radcliffe NHS Trust, Oxford OX3 9DU

Clinical tutor in medicine Nuffield Department of Clinical Medicine, University of Oxford, Oxford

Director of research and development Anglia and Oxford Regional Health Authority, Milton Keynes

Professor of medicine and clinical epidemiology McMaster University, Hamilton, Ontario Canada

Clinical associate professor of medicine University of Rochester School of Medicine and Dentistry, Rochester, New York, USA

David L Sackett, William M C Rosenberg, J A Muir Gray, R Brian Haynes, W Scott Richardson

1. British Medical Association. Report of the working party on medical education. London: *BMA*, 1995.
2. Standing Committee on Postgraduate Medical and Dental Education. Creating a better learning environment in hospitals. 1. Teaching hospital doctors and dentists to teach. London: *SCOPME*, 1994.
3. General Medical Council. Education committee report. London: *GMC*, 1994.
4. Grahame-Smith D. Evidence based medicine: Socratic dissent. *BMJ* 1995;**310**:1126–7.
5. Evidence based medicine; in its place [editorial]. *Lancet* 1995;**346**:785.
6. Correspondence. Evidence based medicine. *Lancet* 1995;**346**:1171–2.
7. Weatherall DJ: The inhumanity of medicine. *BMJ* 1994;**309**:1671–2.
8. House of Commons Health Committee. Priority setting in the NHS: purchasing. First report sessions 1994–95. London: HMSO, 1995. (HC 134-1.)
9. Davidoff F, Haynes B, Sackett D, Smith R. Evidence based medicine: a new journal to help doctors identify the information they need. *BMJ* 1995;**310**:1085–6.
10. Sackett DL. Surveys of self-reported reading times of consultants in Oxford, Birmingham, Milton-Keynes, Bristol, Leicester, and Glasgow. In: Rosenberg WMC, Richardson WS, Haynes RB, Sackett DL. *Evidence-based medicine*. London: Churchill Livingstone (in press).
11. Ellis J, Mulligan I, Rowe J, Sackett DL. Inpatient general medicine is evidence based. *Lancet* 1995;**346**:407–10.
12. Bennett RJ, Sackett DL, Haynes RB, Neufeld VR. A controlled trial of teaching critical appraisal of the clinical literature to medical students. *JAMA* 1987;**257**:2451–4.
13. Shin JH, Flaynes RB, Johnston ME. Effect of problem-based, self-directed undergraduate education on life-long learning. *Can Med Assoc J* 1993;**148**:969–76.

Evidence based medicine: an approach to clinical problem-solving

William Rosenberg, *clinical tutor in medicine*,[a] **Anna Donald**, *senior house officer*[b]

[a] Nuffield Department of Clinical Medicine, John Radcliffe Hospital, Oxford OX3 9DU, [b] Public Health and Health Policy, Anglia and Oxford Regional Health Authority, Oxford OX3 7LF

Correspondence to: Dr Rosenberg.

Doctors within the NHS are confronting major changes at work. While we endeavour to improve the quality of health care, junior doctors' hours have been reduced and the emphasis on continuing medical education has increased. We are confronted by a growing body of information, much of it invalid or irrelevant to clinical practice. This article discusses evidence based medicine, a process of turning clinical problems into questions and then systematically locating, appraising, and using contemporaneous research findings as the basis for clinical decisions. The computerisation of bibliographies and the development of software that permits the rapid location of relevant evidence have made it easier for busy clinicians to make best use of the published literature. Critical appraisal can be used to determine the validity and applicability of the evidence, which is then used to inform clinical decisions. Evidence based medicine can be taught to, and practised by, clinicians at all levels of seniority and can be used to close the gulf between good clinical research and clinical practice. In addition it can help to promote self directed learning and teamwork and produce faster and better doctors.

Doctors must cope with a rapidly changing body of relevant evidence and maximise the quality of medical care despite the reduction in junior doctors' working hours and scarce resources. We are deluged with information, and although much of it is either invalid or irrelevant to clinical practice, an increasing amount comes from powerful investigations such as randomised controlled trials. Yet we continue to base our clinical decisions on increasingly out of date primary training or the overinterpretation of experiences with individual patients,[1] and even dramatically positive results from rigorous clinical studies remain largely unapplied.[2] Doctors need new skills to track down the new types of strong and useful evidence, distinguish it from weak and irrelevant evidence, and put it into practice. In this paper we discuss evidence based medicine, a new framework for clinical problem solving which may help clinicians to meet these challenges.

What is evidence based medicine?

Evidence based medicine is the process of systematically finding, appraising, and using contemporaneous research findings as the basis for clinical decisions. For decades people have been aware of the gaps between research evidence and clinical practice, and the consequences in terms of expensive, ineffective, or even harmful decision making.[3][4] Inexpensive electronic databases and widespread computer literacy now give doctors access to enormous amounts of data. Evidence based medicine is about asking questions, finding and appraising the relevant data, and harnessing that information for everyday clinical practice.

Originally published in *BMJ* 1995; **310**: 1122–6.

Most readers will recognise that the ideas underlying evidence based medicine are not new. Clinicians identify the questions raised in caring for their patients and consult the literature at least occasionally, if not routinely. The difference with using an explicit, evidence based medicine framework is twofold: it can make consulting and evaluating the literature a relatively simple, routine procedure, and it can make this process workable for clinical teams, as well as for individual clinicians. The term "evidence based medicine" was coined at McMaster Medical School in Canada in the 1980s to label this clinical learning strategy, which people at the school had been developing for over a decade.[5]

EVIDENCE BASED MEDICINE IN PRACTICE

Evidence based medicine can be practised in any situation where there is doubt about an aspect of clinical diagnosis, prognosis, or management.

```
Four steps in evidence based medicine
* Formulate a clear clinical question from a patient's
problem
* Search the literature for relevant clinical articles
* Evaluate (critically appraise) the evidence for its
validity and usefulness
* Implement useful findings in clinical practice
```

Setting the question

A 77 year old woman living alone is admitted with non-rheumatic atrial fibrillation and her first bout of mild left ventricular failure, and she responds to digoxin and diuretics. She has a history of well controlled hypertension. An echocardiogram shows moderately impaired left ventricular function. She is an active person and anxious to maintain her independence. During the ward round on the following day a debate ensues about the risks and benefits of offering her long term anticoagulation with warfarin, and rather than defer to seniority or abdicate responsibility to consensus by committee, team members convert the debate into a question: "How does her risk of embolic stroke, if we don't give her anticoagulant drugs, compare with her risk of serious haemorrhage and stroke if we do?"

The questions that initiate evidence based medicine can relate to diagnosis, prognosis, treatment, iatrogenic harm, quality of care, or health economics. In any event, they should be as specific as possible, including the type of patient, the clinical intervention, and the clinical outcome of interest. In this example two questions are prepared for a literature search. One question relates to prognosis and her susceptibility: "How great is the annual risk of embolic stroke in a 77 year old woman with non-rheumatic atrial fibrillation, hypertension, and moderate left ventricular enlargement if she is not given anticoagulants?" The other question concerns treatment and asks, "What is the risk reduction for stroke from warfarin therapy in such a patient, and what is the risk of harming her with this therapy?"

Finding the evidence

The second step is a search for the best available evidence. To conduct searches on a regular basis, clinicians need effective searching skills and easy access to bibliographic databases. Increasingly the access can be proved by ward or surgery based computers, complemented by assistance in obtaining hard copies of articles, and enabled by librarians who teach searching skills and guide the unwary through the 25000 biomedical journals now in print.[6][7]

Two sorts of electronic databases are available. The first sort is bibliographic and permits users to identify relevant citations in the clinical literature, using variations of Medline. The second sort of database takes the user directly to primary or secondary publications of the relevant clinical evidence — the rapidly growing numbers include the Cochrane Database of Systematic Reviews, Scientific American Medicine on CD-ROM, and the ACP Journal Club (a bimonthly supplement to the Annals of Internal Medicine which abstracts the relevant and rigorous articles on diagnosis, prognosis, treatment, quality of care, and medical economics from over 30 general medical journals). All these databases are, or soon will be, available on line from local, national, and international networks such as the internet.

For our patient, the searches were conducted with Medline and the Knowledge Finder searching software. "Atrial fibrillation" and "cerebrovascular disorders" were entered as major medical subject headings and "randomised controlled trial" as a publication type selected from the "dictionaries" menu. The search was performed twice, once with "prognosis" entered as a freetext search parameter and a second time with "therapy" included. The years 1990-4 were searched and 10 articles were identified, of which eight seemed to contain the relevant information (two on prognosis[8 9] and six reporting randomised trials of therapy[10 11 12 13 14 15]). Five[10 11 12 13 14] were available in the library.

The search was repeated for 1992-4 with "review" as the publication type, and one recent article was identified.[16] The term "review" includes subjective reviews, systematic reviews, and meta-analyses. The newer term "meta-analysis" could have been used as a publication type to narrow the search but would have missed potentially useful reviews and systematic reviews, as well as meta-analyses that have not yet been classified as such in Medline.

The two articles on prognosis, four on therapy, and the review (in fact a meta-analysis) were then pulled from the library. The keyboard time taken for this search was 15 minutes. The ACP Journal Club, whose electronic version is currently being tested, has summarised these trials, and Cochrane reviews on the prevention and treatment of stroke will be available in 1995, but on this occasion we examined the evidence presented in conventional forms of clinical research publication.

While clinicians may make greater use of meta-analyses in the future, the ability to appraise critically publications of all types will remain an invaluable skill. Searches may fail to uncover well conducted and relevant meta-analyses and often it will be impractical for a busy clinician to conduct an independent systematic review of the literature each time a clinical question is generated. On these occasions the most effective strategy will be to seek out the best of the available literature and to appraise critically the evidence by using skills that can readily be learnt.

Appraising the evidence

The third step is to evaluate, or appraise, the evidence for its validity and clinical usefulness. This step is crucial because it lets the clinician decide whether an article can be relied on to give useful guidance. Unfortunately, a large proportion of published medical research lacks either relevance or sufficient methodological rigour to be reliable enough for answering clinical questions.[17] To overcome this, a structured but simple method, named "critical appraisal," developed by several teams working in North America and the United Kingdom, enables individuals without research expertise to evaluate clinical articles. Mastering critical appraisal entails learning how to ask a few key questions about the validity of the evidence and its relevance to a particular patient or group of patients. Its fundamentals can be learnt within a few hours in small tutorials, workshops, interactive lectures, and at the bedside by a wide range of users, including those without a biomedical background. This strategy has been developed for many different types of articles, and can be used to evaluate original articles about diagnosis, treatment, prognosis, quality of care, and economics as well as to evaluate reviews, overviews, and meta-analyses for their validity and applicability.

The table shows a typical set of critical appraisal questions for evaluating articles about treatment. Although they reflect common sense, the questions are not entirely self explanatory; some instruction is needed to help clinicians apply them to specific articles and individual patients. Self directed learning materials have been developed to help users apply different critical appraisal questions to the different sorts of clinical research articles on diagnosis, prognosis, therapy, quality of care, economic analysis, and screening. These materials include the JAMA series of user's guides and the text *Clinical Epidemiology: A Basic Science for Clinical Medicine*.[18] Week long training workshops in evidence based medicine are held in various venues, but we have found that even people with limited experience can readily learn how to practise evidence based medicine in the context of their own clinical practice. As with any other skill, expertise and speed come with practice, and experienced practitioners can learn to appraise critically most articles in under 10 minutes, transforming themselves from passive, opinion based spectators to active, evidence based clinicians.

```
Critical appraisal questions used to evaluate a therapy article[19] [20]
-----------------------------------------------------------------------
                                              Yes     Can't tell     No
-----------------------------------------------------------------------
Are the results valid?
  Was the assignment of patients to
    treatments randomised?
  Were all patients who entered the trial
    properly accounted for and
    attributed at its conclusion?
      Was follow up complete?
      Were patients analysed in the groups to
        which they were randomised?
  Were patients, health workers, and study
    personnel blinded to treatment?
  Were the groups similar at the start of the trial?
  Aside from the experimental intervention,
    were the groups treated equally?
What are the results?
  How large was the treatment effect?
  How precise was the treatment effect?
Will the results help me care for my patients?
  Can the results be applied to my patient care?
  Were all clinically important outcomes
    considered?
  Are the likely benefits worth the potential
    harms and costs?
```

This transformation is borne out in the critical appraisal of the evidence surrounding the management of the 77 year old woman with atrial fibrillation. The two articles on prognosis fulfil criteria for validity and applicability and reveal that our particular patient faces an 18% annual risk of stroke if left untreated.[8] [9] Applying criteria given in the Users' guides to the medical literature: how to use an article about therapy or prevention,[19] [20] we decided that the articles we have pulled provide valid and applicable evidence. We used them to obtain the relative risk reduction of stroke due to treatment with warfarin, which is 70%. The annual risk of stroke for our patient without treatment was used, in conjunction with relative risk reduction obtained from the prognosis articles, to calculate the absolute risk reduction (ARR) of stroke attributable to anticoagulation with warfarin. This figure, which is 0.13, was then used to calculate the "number needed to treat" (NNT=1/ARR) with warfarin to save one stroke. Thus treating eight patients (1/0.13) for one year will prevent one stroke. The annual rate of major haemorrhage in patients receiving warfarin is 1%, so one patient in every hundred taking warfarin will experience a major bleed each year, and we therefore can expect to prevent about 13 strokes in patients such as ours with warfarin for every major bleed we will cause through such treatment. Although the benefit:risk ratio seems acceptable in this instance, we know that bleeding rates vary between centres and a higher local risk of intracranial haemorrhage might lead other clinicians and patients to a very different decision. The evidence will not automatically dictate patient care but will provide the factual basis on which decisions can be made, taking all aspects of patient care into consideration.

Acting on the evidence

Having identified evidence that is both valid and relevant, clinicians can either implement it directly in a patient's care or use it to develop team protocols or even hospital guidelines. They can also use evidence to revolutionise continuing medical education programmes or audit. In our experience, implementing the evidence is best learned through group discussions, either on ward rounds or in other meetings of the clinical team in which members explore ways of incorporating the evidence into a patient's clinical management.

At the weekly firm meeting the evidence extracted from the critically appraised literature on warfarin was presented in a summarised form as a critically appraised topic by a junior member of the team (table). During the subsequent ward round the team discussed the evidence with the patient and she decided to start taking warfarin. It was decided to set a target international normalised ratio of 1.5-2.0, and her general practitioner, who asked for a copy of the critically appraised topic to accompany the discharge letter, agreed to monitor her treatment.

OTHER REQUIREMENTS FOR PRACTISING EVIDENCE BASED MEDICINE

Clear data presentation

The ability to present published evidence quickly and clearly is crucial for clinical teams with little time and much information to absorb.[21] Medical journals have led the way here with structured abstracts to help readers quickly retrieve key information. Such clarity and quickness are equally important for clinicians when they present evidence to their team. A preset, one page, user friendly summary such as the one developed by doctors in training at McMaster University in Ontario (unpublished data) can help this process and was the model for the critically appraised topic that appears in the table.

```
Added advantages in practising evidence
based medicine
For individuals
* Enables clinicians to upgrade their knowledge base
routinely
* Improves clinicians' understanding of research
methods and makes them more critical in using data
* Improves confidence in management decisions
* Improves computer literacy and data searching
techniques
* Improves reading habits
For clinical teams
* Gives team a framework for group problem solving
and for teaching
* Enables juniors to contribute usefully to team
For patients
* More effective use of resources
* Better communication with patients about the
rationale behind management decisions
```

Senior support

Support from senior clinicians is critical to the success of introducing evidence based medicine.[22] Seniors who practice evidence based medicine are excellent role models for training newcomers and allocating questions according to the skills and time commitments of individual team members. Even when senior staff are themselves unfamiliar with evidence based medicine, their willingness to admit uncertainty, to encourage scepticism, and to be flexible can help the team to accommodate new evidence which may contradict previous assumptions and practice.

DOES IT WORK?

An evidence based approach to clinical care has been practised in many countries under various guises. In the structured form described above it attracts both support and criticism, often within the same hospital. The problem, ironically, is that the approach is difficult to evaluate.[23] It is a process for solving problems, and it will have different outcomes depending on the problem being solved. Trying to monitor all the possible outcomes would be impossible, especially since many are difficult to quantify. For example, a medical student who learns the importance of good research methodology through practising critical appraisal may later on carry out better research, but it would be hard either to quantify this or to link it directly to evidence based medicine.

None the less, evidence of the effectiveness of evidence based medicine is growing as it spreads to new settings. Short term trials have shown better and more informed clinical decisions following even brief training in critical appraisal,[24] and although graduates from traditional medical curriculums progressively decline in their knowledge of appropriate clinical practice, graduates of a medical school that teaches lifelong, self directed, evidence based medicine are still up to date as long as 15 years after graduation.[25] The review of the benefits and drawbacks of evidence based medicine that follows draws on our experience of teaching and practising evidence based medicine with clinicians and purchasers in Oxford.

ADVANTAGES

An immediate attraction of evidence based medicine is that it integrates medical education with clinical practice. We have observed that students and doctors who begin to learn evidence based medicine become adept at generating their own questions and following them through with efficient literature searches. For example, learners quickly learn to pick out good review articles and to use resources such as the ACP Journal Club when they are appropriate to the question being asked.[26]

Another advantage of evidence based medicine is that it can be learnt by people from different backgrounds and at any stage in their careers. Medical students carrying out critical appraisals not only learn evidence based medicine for themselves but contribute their appraisals to their teams and update their colleagues. At the other extreme, seasoned clinicians can master evidence based medicine and transform a journal club from a passive summary of assigned journals into an active inquiry in which problems arising from patient care are used to direct searches and appraisals of relevant evidence to keep their practice up to date.

The evidence based approach is being taken up by non-clinicians as well. Consumer groups concerned with obtaining optimal care during pregnancy and childbirth are evolving evidence based patient choice. The critical appraisal skills for purchasers project in the former Oxford region involves teaching evidence based medicine to purchasers who have no medical training so that it can inform their decisions on purchasing.[27]

A third attraction of evidence based medicine is its potential for improving continuity and uniformity of care through the common approaches and guidelines developed by its practitioners. Shift work and cross cover make communication between health workers both more important and more difficult. Although evidence based medicine cannot alter work relationships, in our experience it does provide a structure for effective team work and the open communication of team generated (rather than externally imposed) guidelines for optimal patient care. It also provides a common framework for problem solving and improving communication and understanding between people from different backgrounds, such as clinicians and patients or non-medical purchasers and clinicians.

Evidence based medicine can help providers make better use of limited resources by enabling them to evaluate clinical effectiveness of treatments and services. Remaining ignorant of valid research findings has serious consequences. For example, it is now clear that giving steroids to women at risk of premature labour greatly reduces infant respiratory distress and consequent morbidity, mortality, and costs of care,[28] and it is equally clear that aspirin and streptokinase deserve to be among the mainstays of care for victims of heart attack.

DISADVANTAGES

Evidence based medicine has several drawbacks. Firstly, it takes time both to learn and to practise. For example, it takes about two hours to properly set the question, find the evidence, appraise the evidence, and act on the evidence, and for teams to benefit all members should be present for the first and last steps. Senior staff must therefore be good at time management. They can help to make searches less onerous by setting achievable contracts with the team members doing the searches and by ensuring that the question has direct clinical usefulness. These responsibilities of the team leader are time consuming.

Establishing the infrastructure for practising evidence based medicine costs money. Hospitals and general practices may need to buy and maintain the necessary computer hardware and software. CD-ROM subscriptions can vary from pounds sterling 250 to pounds sterling 2000 a year, depending on the database and specifications. But a shortage of resources need not stifle the adoption of evidence based medicine. The BMA provides Medline free of charge to members with modems, and Medline is also available for a small fee on the internet. Compared with the costs of many medical interventions (to say nothing of journal subscriptions and out of date texts), these costs are small and may recover costs many times their amount by reducing ineffective practice.

Inevitably, evidence based medicine exposes gaps in the evidence.[4] This can be frustrating, particularly for inexperienced doctors. Senior staff can help to overcome this problem by setting questions for which there is likely to be good evidence. The identification of such gaps can be helpful in generating local and national research projects, such as those being commissioned by the York Centre for Reviews and Dissemination.[29]

Another problem is that Medline and the other electronic databases used for finding relevant evidence are not comprehensive and are not always well indexed. At times even a lengthy literature search is fruitless. For some older doctors the computer skills needed for using databases regularly may also seem daunting. Although the evidence based approach requires a minimum of computer literacy and keyboard skills, and while these are now almost universal among medical students and junior doctors, many older doctors are still unfamiliar with computers and databases. On the other hand, creative and systematic searching techniques are increasingly available, [30] [33] and high quality review articles are becoming abundant. In the absence of suitcal review articles, clinicians who have acquired critical appraisal skills will be able to evaluate the primary literature for themselves.

Finally, authoritarian clinicians may see evidence based medicine as a threat. It may cause them to lose face by sometimes exposing their current practice as obsolete or occasionally even dangerous. At times it will alter the dynamics of the team, removing hierarchical distinctions that are based on seniority; some will rue the day when a junior member of the team, by conducting a search and critical appraisal, has as much authority and respect as the team's most senior member.[32]

We thank the following for their advice and support: John Bell, Muir Gray, Ruairidh Milne, Anne Lusher, Fiona Godlee, Brian Haynes, Val Lawrence, David Sackett, Sir David Weatherall.

William Rosenberg is supported by a grant from the Department of Health's undergraduate medical curriculum implementation support scheme.

1. Smith R. Filling the lacuna between research and practice: an interview with Michael Peckham. *BMJ* 1993;**307**:1403–7.
2. Faber RG. Information overload. *BMJ* 1993;**307**:383.
3. Haines A, Jones R. Implementing findings of research. *BMJ* 1994;**308**:1488–92.
4. Chalmers I, Dickersin K, Chalmers TC. Getting to grips with Archie Cochrane's agenda. *BMJ* 1992;**305**:786–7.
5. Evidence Based Medicine Working Group. Evidence based medicine. *JAMA* 1992;**268**:2420–5.
6. Wyatt J. Uses and sources of medical knowledge. *Lancet* 1991;**338**:1368–73.
7. Marshall JG. The impact of the hospital library on clinical decision making: the Rochester study. *Bulletin of the Medical Library Association* 1992;**80**:169–78.
8. SPAF Investigators. Predictors of thromboembolism in atrial fibrillation. I. Clinical features in patients at risk. *Ann Intern Med* 1992;**116**:1–5.
9. SPAF Investigators. Predicators of thromboembolism in atrial fibrillation. II. Echocardiographic features in patients at risk. *Ann Intern Med* 1992;**116**:6–12.
10. Petersen P, Boysen G, Godtfredsen J, Andersen ED, Andersen B. Placebo controlled randomised trial of warfarin and aspirin for the prevention of thromboembolic complications in chronic atrial fibrillation. *Lancet* 1989;**i**:175–9.
11. Boston Area Anticoagulation Trial for Atrial Fibrillation Investigators. The effect of low-dose warfarin on the risk of stroke in patients with non-rheumatic atrial fibrillation. *N Engl J Med* 1990;**323**:1505–11.
12. Stroke Prevention in Atrial Fibrillation Investigators. Stroke prevention in atrial fibrillation study: final results. *Circulation* 1991;**84**:527–39.
13. Ezekowitz MD, Bridgers L, James KE, Carliner NH, Colling CL, Gomick CC, *et al.* Warfarin in the prevention of stroke associated with non-rheumatic atrial fibrillation. *N Engl J Med* 1992;**347**:1406–12.
14. Stroke Prevention in Atrial Fibrillation Investigators. Warfarin versus aspirin for prevention of thromboembolism in atrial fibrillation: stroke prevention in atrial fibrillation II study. *Lancet*, **343**:687–91.
15. Connolly SJ, Laupacis A, Gent M, Roberts RS, Cairns JA, Joyner C. Candian atrial fibrillation anticoagulation (CAFA) study. *J Am Coll Cardiol* 1991;**18**:349–55.
16. Atrial Fibrillation Investigators. Risk factors for stroke and efficacy of antithrombotic therapy in atrial fibrillation: analysis of pooled data from randomised controlled trials. *Arch Intern Med* 1994;**154**:1449–57.
17. Altman DG. The scandal of poor medical research. *BMJ* 1994;**308**:283–4.

18. Sackett DL, Haynes RB, Guyatt GH, Tugwell P. *Clinical epidemiology: a basic science for clinical medicine*. 2nd ed. Boston: Little, Brown, 1991.

19. Users' guides to the medical literature: how to use an article about therapy or prevention. I. *JAMA* 1993;**270**:2598–601.

20. Users guides to the medical literature: how to use an article about therapy or prevention. II. *JAMA* 1994;**271**:59–63.

21. Lock S. Structured abstracts. *BMJ* 1988;**297**:156.

22. Guyatt G, Nishikawa J. A proposal for enhancing the quality of clinical teaching: results of a department of medicine's educational retreat. *Medical Teacher* 1993;**15**:147–61.

23. Audet N, Gagnon R, Marcil M. L'enseignement de l'analyse critique des publications scientifiques medicales, est-il efficace? Revision des études et de leur qualité methodologique. *Can Med Assoc J* 1993;**148**:945–52.

24. Bennet KJ, Sackett DL, Haynes RB, Neufeld VR. A controlled trial of teaching critical appraisal of the clinical literature to medical students. *JAMA* 1987;**257**:2451–4.

25. Shin JH, Haynes RB, Johnson ME. The effect of problem-based, self-directed undergraduate education on life-long learning. *Can Med Assoc J* 1993;**148**:969–76.

26. Milne R, Chambers L. Assessing the scientific quality of review articles. *J Epidemiol Community Health* 1993;**47**:169–70.

27. Dunning M, McQuay H, Milne R. Getting a GRiP. *Health Service Journal* 1994;**104**:24–6.

28. Crowley P, Chalmers I, Keirse MJ. The effects of corticosteroid administration before pre-term delivery: an overview of the evidence from controlled trials. *Br J Object Gynaecol* 1990;**97**:11–25.

29. Sheldon T, Chalmers I. The UK Cochrane Centre and the NHS Centre for Reviews and Dissemination: respective roles within the information systems strategy of the NHS R&D programme, co-ordination and principles underlying collaboration. *Health Economics* 1994;**3**:201–3.

30. Farbey R. Searching the literature: be creative with Medline. *BMJ* 1993;**307**:66.

31. Jadad AR, McQuay H. Searching the literature: be systematic in your searching. *BMJ* 1993;**307**:66.

32. West R. Assessment of evidence versus consensus or prejudice. *J Epidemiol Community Health* 1993;**47**:321–2.

"Is my practice evidence based?"

Should be answered in qualitative, as well as quantitative terms.

The growing interest in evidence based medicine among practising clinicians[1] has prompted doctors in every specialty to ask themselves, "to what extent is the care of my patients evidence based?" The search is on for a means of answering this question that is achievable, affordable, valid, reliable, and responsive to change.

Evaluating one's own performance is the final step in the five stage process of traditional evidence based practice. The first four steps are: to formulate for each chosen clinical problem an answerable question, to search the medical literature and other sources for information pertaining to that question, to assess the validity (closeness to the truth) and usefulness (relevance to the problem) of the evidence identified, and to manage the patient accordingly.[2]

Several papers have been published[3][4][5] and many more are being written whose stated objective is "to assess whether my/our clinical practice is evidence based." Most describe prospective surveys of a consecutive series of doctor-patient encounters in a particular specialty, in which the primary intervention for each patient was classified by the doctors (and in some cases verified by an independent observer) according to whether it was based on evidence from randomised controlled trials, convincing non-experimental evidence, or inadequate evidence.

Such surveys have generated the widely quoted figures that 82% of interventions in general medicine,[3] 81% of interventions in general practice,[4] and 62% of interventions in psychiatry[5] are evidence based. Questionnaire surveys of what doctors say they do in particular circumstances are starting to add to this literature.[6] The public may soon be offered a "league table" of specialties ranked according to how evidence based they have shown themselves to be.

Figures produced in the early 1980s suggested that only about 15% of medical practice was based on sound scientific evidence.[7] Is the spate of new studies, therefore, grounds for reassurance that medical practice has become dramatically more evidence based in the past 15 years? Probably not. The earlier estimates were derived by assessing all diagnostic and therapeutic procedures currently in use, so that each procedure, however obscure, carried equal weight in the final figure. A more recent evaluation using this method classified 21% of health technologies as evidence based.[8] The latest surveys, which looked at interventions chosen for real patients, were designed with the laudable objective of assessing the technologies which were actually used rather than simply those that are on the market.

But the impressive percentages obtained in these series should be interpreted cautiously. As the protagonists of evidence based medicine themselves have taught us, a survey of any aspect of medical care should, in order to be generalisable beyond the particular sample studied, meet criteria for representativeness (are the health professionals and patients described typical?), data collection (is the sample unbiased?), data analysis (were all potential subjects included in the denominator or otherwise accounted for, and was assessment "blind"?), validity (were appropriate criteria used to

Originally published in *BMJ* 1996; **313**: 957–8.

classify subjects, and were these criteria applied rigorously?), comprehensiveness (was the study large enough and complete enough to make the results credible?), and repeatability (would the same results be obtained if the sample were studied on another occasion?).[2]

```
Is my practice evidence based? A context specific
checklist for individual clinical encounters

Have you
1 Identified and prioritised the clinical, psychological, social, and
other problems, taking into account the patient's perspective?
2 Performed a sufficiently competent and complete examination to
establish the likelihood of competing diagnoses?
3 Considered additional problems and risk factors?
4 Where necessary, sought relevant evidence--from systematic
reviews, guidelines, clinical trials, and other sources?
5 Assessed and taken into account the completeness, quality, and
strength of the evidence, and its relevance to this patient?
6 Presented the pros and cons of the different options to the
patient in a way they can understand, and incorporated the
patient's utilities into the final recommendations?
```

A survey which addressed the question "Is my practice evidence-based?" and which fulfilled all these criteria would be a major and highly expensive undertaking. But even if it were practically possible, several theoretical limitations would remain. The most important of these is that patients rarely enter the consulting room (or the operating theatre) with a discrete, one dimensional problem. A study which, for good practical reasons, looks at one clinical decision per case necessarily reduces the complexities of each patient's wants and needs to a single decision node. Such an approach might occasionally come close to being valid, but many aspects of management in primary care,[9] care of older people,[10] and chronic medical conditions[11] do not lend themselves to the formulation of single answerable questions or the application of discrete, definitive interventions. In general practice, for example, the usual diagnostic and therapeutic sequence of diagnosis by epidemiological classification–symptoms and signs leading to identification of the disease, leading to treatment–may be less appropriate than diagnosis by prognosis–symptoms and signs leading to a provisional hypothesis, leading to watchful waiting, leading to identification of the disease–or diagnosis by therapeutic response–symptoms and signs leading to a provisional hypothesis, leading to empirical treatment, leading to identification of the disease.[2]

Failure to recognise the legitimacy of these variations in approach has created a somewhat spurious divide between those who seek to establish general practice on an equal "scientific" footing to that of the secondary care sector[4][12] and those who emphasise the value of the intuitive, narrative, and interpretive aspects of the consultation.[13] Others have argued that both "science" and "art" are essential elements of evidence based care, which strives to integrate the best external evidence with all round clinical expertise.[1][14] Nevertheless, debate continues as to whether all round clinical expertise can be dissected down to a set of objective and measurable components that are amenable to formal performance review[15] or whether it is ultimately subjective and one of the unsolvable mysteries of the art of medicine.[16]

Perhaps the most difficult aspect of evidence based practice to evaluate is the extent to which the evidence, insofar as it exists, has been applied with due regard to the personal priorities of the patient being treated.[17] It is said that this step can be made objective by incorporating the weighted preferences of patients (utilities) into a decision tree.[18] But researchers have found that defining and measuring the degree of patient centredness of a medical decision is a methodological minefield.[19]

Here lies the real challenge of evidence based practice. Randomised controlled trials may constitute the ideal of experimental design, but they alone cannot prove that the right intervention has been provided to the right patient at the right time and place. To show that a decision on drug treatment was evidence based, for example, it is not sufficient to cite a single randomised controlled trial (or meta-analysis of several similar trials) in which the drug was shown to be more effective than placebo. It must also be shown that the prescriber defined the ultimate objective of treatment (such as cure, prevention of later complications, palliation, or reassurance) and selected the most appropriate treatment using all available evidence. This decision requires consideration of whether a different drug, or no drug, would suit the patient better, and whether the so called "treatment of choice" is viewed as such by the patient.[2]

To seek, through scientific inquiry, an honest and objective assessment of how far we are practising evidence based medicine is an exercise which few of us would dare embark on. But research studies designed to address this question via the methodology of traditional "process of care" audit[3 4 5 6] inform the doctor of a limited aspect of his or her efforts. In measuring what is most readily measurable, they reduce the multidimensional doctor-patient encounter to a bald dichotomy ("the management of this case was/was not evidence based") and may thereby distort rather than summarise the doctor's overall performance.

Measuring every dimension of care in a large consecutive series of cases would be impossible. It is surely time that we eschewed the inherent reductionism of audit by numbers and tried to capture more context in our reviews of clinical performance. Issues that are complex, multidimensional, and grounded in individual experience lend themselves to study by descriptive and qualitative methods.[20] At the very least, future attempts to answer the question "how evidence based is my practice?" should include some measure of how competing clinical questions were prioritised for each case and how the evidence obtained was particularised to reflect the needs and choices of the individual patient.

I thank Professor Ann-Louise Kinmonth and the members of the evidence-based-health mailbase on the Internet for valuable comments on earlier drafts of this manuscript.

Trisha Greenhalgh, Senior lecturer

Joint Department of Primary Care and Population Sciences, University College London Medical School/Royal Free Hospital School of Medicine, Whittington Hospital, London N19 5NF

Trisha Greenhalgh

1. Sackett DL, Rosenberg WMC, Gray JAM, Haynes RB, Richardson WS. Evidence-based medicine: what is it and what isn't it. *BMJ* 1996;**312**:71–2.
2. Sackett DL, Haynes RB, Guyatt GH, Tugwell P. *Clinical epidemiology–a basic science for clinical medicine*. London: Little, Brown, 1991: 187.
3. Ellis J, Mulligan I, Rowe J, Sackett DL. Inpatient general medicine is evidence-based. A-team, Nuffield Department of Clinical Medicine. *Lancet* 1995;**345**:407–10.
4. Gill P, Dowell AC, Neal RD, Smith N, Heywood P, Wilson AF. Evidence based general practice: a retrospective study of interventions in one training practice. *BMJ* 1996;**312**:812–21.
5. Geddes J, Game D, Jenkins N, Peterson LA, Pottinger GR, Sackett DL. *In patient psychiatric treatment is evidence-based*. Qual Health Care (in press).
6. Little P, Smith L, Cantrell T, Chapman J, Langridge J, Pickering R. General practitioners' management of acute back pain, a survey of reported practice compares with clinical guidelines. *BMJ* 1996;**312**:485–8.

7. Office of Technology Assessment of the Congress of the United States. The impact of randomised clinical trials on health policy and medical practice. Washington DC: US Government Printing Office, 1983.
8. Dubinsky M, Ferguson JH. Analysis of the National Institutes of Health Medicare coverage assessment. *Int J Technol Assess Health Care* 1990;**6**:480–8.
9. Charlton R. Balancing science and art in primary care research: past and present. *Br J Gen Pract* 1995;**45**:639–40.
10. Grimley Evans J. Evidence-based and evidence biased medicine. *Age Ageing* 1995;**25**:461–4.
11. Naylor CD. Gray zones of clinical practice: some limits to evidence-based medicine. *Lancet* 1995;**345**:840–2.
12. Dawes MG. On the need for evidence-based general and family practice. *Evidence-Based Med* 1996;**1**:68–9.
13. Smith BH, Taylor RJ. *Medicine–a healing or a dying art? Br J Gen Pract* 1996;**46**:249–51.
14. Slawson DC, Shaughnessy AF, Bennett JH. Becoming a medical information master, feeling good about not knowing everything. *J Fam Pract* 1994;**28**:505–13.
15. Sackett DL, Rennie D. The science of the art of the clinical examination. *JAMA* 1992;**267**:650–2.
16. Tannenbaum SJ. What physicians know. *N Engl J Med* 1993;**329**:1268–71.
17. Haynes RB, Hayward RS, Lomas J. Bridges between health care research evidence and clinical practice. *J Am Med Inf Assoc* 1995;**2**:342–50.
18. Kassirer JP. Incorporating patients' preferences into medical decisions. *N Engl J Med* 1994;**330**:1895–6.
19. Blaxter M. *Consumers and research in the NHS; consumer issues within the NHS.* Leeds: Department of Health Publications, 1994. (Report No G60/002 2954.)
20. Kinmonth A-L. Understanding and meaning in research and practice. *Fam Pract* 1995;**12**:1–2.

BMJ

Medicine based evidence, a prerequisite for evidence based medicine

Future research methods must find ways of accommodating clinical reality, not ignoring it

Seeking an evidence base for medicine is as old as medicine itself, but in the past decade the concept of evidence based medicine has done a good job in focusing explicit attention on the application of evidence from valid clinical research to clinical practice.[1] [2] Although current clinical practice is often evidence based,[3] [4] there is still much to be gained. Important new evidence from research often takes a long time to be implemented in daily care, while established practices persist even if they have been proved to be ineffective or harmful.[5] In the meantime, many clinicians struggle to apply the results of studies that do not seem that relevant to their daily practice.

Evidence based medicine has been defined as the "conscientious, explicit and judicious use of current best evidence in making decisions about the care of individual patients."[2] What can we learn from the limitations of current best evidence for the way that we design future studies?

We face the problem that criteria for internal and external validity (that is, clinical applicability) may conflict. Clinical studies are usually performed on a homogeneous study population and exclude clinically complex cases for the sake of internal validity. Such selection may not, however, match the type of patients for whom the studied intervention will be considered. Medical practice is often confronted with patients presenting several problems.[6] [7] Older patients and women are under-represented in clinical trials,[8] [9] and patients with comorbidity, a common phenomenon at older ages,[10] are generally excluded. Evidence from patients selected by referral cannot easily be generalised to patients seen in primary care with less severe or early stage clinical pictures.[6] And some important needs for evidence are almost ignored. For instance, while drug trials usually provide evidence about starting drug treatment, doctors are increasingly confronted by patients taking multiple long term medications but have no proper data on evidence based drug cessation.

Studies on the effectiveness of clinical care may also not easily attain internal validity. An example is the evaluation of the many interventions that cannot be blinded, such as many non-pharmacological procedures. Then, to avoid methodological calamities such as contamination of trial arms, choices must be made between not evaluating at all or looking for alternative design options such as pre-randomisation.[11] In studying the effects of complex clinical guidelines the problems are even greater. In addition, the evaluation of diagnostic procedures struggles with difficulties often not dealt with in methodological textbooks. For instance, in validating diagnostic information on low back pain, chronic fatigue syndrome, and benign prostatic hyperplasia unequivocal "gold standard" procedures or even concepts do not exist. And for symptoms and signs such as chronic abdominal pain or a raised erythrocyte sedimentation rate[12] invasive gold standard procedures cannot be routinely carried out. Current best evidence may then come from "delayed type cross sectional studies" that harvest the reference standard information from a thorough clinical follow up. Such solutions may not be ideal but the best achievable, closely connected with the reality of clinical care.

Originally published in *BMJ* 1997; **315**: 1109–10.

Thus, in seeking internally valid evidence that is externally valid for clinical practice, we need "medicine based" studies that include, not ignore, clinical reality and its inherent difficulties. Since no individual study can include full clinical reality, meta-analyses of various diagnostic and therapeutic studies including various relevant subgroups (such as elderly patients[13] or those with comorbidity) are indispensable. To support individual decision making, these meta-analyses should evaluate effect modification between subgroups rather than seeking overall effect measures adjusted for subgroup differences. In (inter)national collaborations such evidence can be prospectively collected, but many methodological problems remain to be resolved, such as cultural differences in symptom perception and therapeutic traditions.

In reviewing clinical evidence we must be reluctant to adopt too detailed criteria for good and bad science and to freeze criteria for validity. Study methods themselves need to evolve. The randomised controlled trial was developed over half a century and refined in the slipstream of important clinical questions, rather than the reverse. At the same time, much knowledge gained before randomised controlled trials came into being survived into the era of the randomised controlled trial. Given the limited coverage of clinical practice by questions susceptible to randomised controlled trials, quasi-experimental methods that respect the principle of comparability may grow more important—for example, in comparing procedures more or less allocated by chance in daily practice, with negligible confounding by indication. Power requirements for individual studies may become less critical in an era of prospective accumulation of evidence. Databases and practice computer networks will provide for a continuum, from evidence from individual practice to collaborative sampling frames for clinical research.[14] In promoting such processes the clinical community can capitalise on the natural interaction between practice (with learning from informal evidence) and clinical research designs (in order to learn formally) (see box).

Relation between clinical practice and clinical research designs

Clinical practice	*Appropriate design for clinical research*
Exploration of hypotheses	Qualitative research
History taking	Case-control study
Diagnostic testing	Cross sectional study
Treatment experience	Randomised clinical trial
Individual trial and error	n of 1 trial
Following clinical course	Cohort study
Record keeping	Systematic registry based (computer supported) research
Individual peer review	Quality of care research/process evaluation

---

Finally, in using strict criteria in reviewing manuscripts for publication, we should worry about risk avoidance by clinical researchers. They might focus their energies on topics where the methodological criteria of reviewers and editors can be most easily met, rather than studying real life clinical problems which present substantial methodological problems. Such "criteria bias" is to be prevented, since medicine based evidence is a prerequisite for evidence based medicine.

Geert Jan Dinant, *Associate professor* [a]

[a] Department of General Practice, Maastricht University, PO Box 616, 6200 MD Maastricht, The Netherlands
Andre.Knottnerus@hagunimaas.nl

1. Evidence-Based Medicine Working Group. Evidence-based medicine: a new approach to teaching the practice of medicine. *JAMA* 1992;**268**:2420–5.
2. Sackett DL, Rosenberg WMC, Gray JAM, Haynes RB, Richardson WS. Evidence based medicine: what it is and what it isn't. It's about integrating individual clinical expertise and the best external evidence. *BMJ* 1996;**312**:71–2.
3. Ellis J, Mulligan, Rowe J, Sackett DL. Inpatient general medicine is evidence-based. A-team, Nuffield Department of Clinical Medicine. *Lancet* 1995;**345**:407–10.
4. Gill P, Dowell AC, Neal RD, Smith N, Heywood P, Wilson AE. Evidence-based general practice: a retrospective study of interventions in one training practice. *BMJ* 1996;**312**:819–21.
5. Martensen RL. The effect of medical conservatism on the acceptance of important medical discoveries. *JAMA* 1996;**276**:1933.
6. Knottnerus JA. Medical decision making by general practitioners and specialists. *Fam Pract* 1991;**8**:305–7.
7. Greenhalgh T. Is my practice evidence-based? Should be answered in qualitative, as well as quantitative terms. *BMJ* 1996;**313**:957–8.
8. Gurwitz JH, Col NF, Avorn J. The exclusion of the elderly and women from clinical trials in acute myocardial infarction. *JAMA* 1992;**268**:1417–22.
9. Trimble EL, Carter CL, Cain D, Freidlin B, Ungerleider R, Friedman M. Representation of older patients in cancer treatment trials. *Cancer* 1994;**74**:2208–14.
10. Schellevis FG, Velden J vd, Lisdonk E vd, Eijk J ThM van, Weel C van. Comorbidity of chronic diseases in general practice. *J Clin Epidemiol* 1993;**46**:469–73.
11. Vierhout WPM, Knottnerus JA, Van Ooij A, Crebolder HFJM, Pop P, Wesselingh-Megens A, *et al*. Effectiveness of joint consultation sessions of general practitioners and orthopaedic surgeons for locomotor system disorders. *Lancet* 1995;**346**:990–4.
12. Dinant GJ, Knottnerus JA, Van Wersch JWJ. Discriminating ability of the erythrocyte sedimentation rate: a prospective study in general practice. *Br J Gen Pract* 1991;**41**:365–70.
13. Rochon PA, Dickinson E, Gordon M. The Cochrane field in health care of older people: geriatric medicine's role in the collaboration. *JAGS* 1997;**45**:241–43.
14. Metsemakers JFM. Unlocking patients' records in general practice for research, medical education and quality assurance: the Registration Network Family Practices [thesis]. Maastricht: Maastricht University, 1994.

Narrative based medicine
Narrative based medicine in an evidence based world

Trisha Greenhalgh

In a widely quoted riposte to critics who accused them of naive empiricism, Sackett and colleagues claimed that "the practice of evidence based medicine means integrating individual clinical expertise with the best available external clinical evidence …. By individual clinical expertise we mean the proficiency and judgment that individual clinicians acquire through clinical experience and clinical practice."[1] Sackett and colleagues were anxious to acknowledge that there is an art to medicine as well as an objective empirical science but they did not attempt to define or categorise the elusive quality of clinical competence. This article explores the dissonance between the "science" of objective measurement[2] and the "art" of clinical proficiency and judgment,[3–5] and attempts to integrate these different perspectives on clinical method.

The limits of objectivity in clinical method

Science is concerned with the formulation and attempted falsification of hypotheses using reproducible methods that allow the construction of generalisable statements about how the universe behaves. Conventional medical training teaches students to view medicine as a science and the doctor as an impartial investigator who builds differential diagnoses as if they were scientific theories and who excludes competing possibilities in a manner akin to the falsification of hypotheses. This approach is based on the somewhat tenuous assumption that diagnostic decision making follows an identical protocol to scientific inquiry—in other words, that the discovery of "facts" about a patient's illness is equivalent to the discovery of new scientific truths about the universe.

The evidence based approach to clinical decision making is often incorrectly held to rest on the assumption that clinical observation is totally objective and should, like all scientific measurements, be reproducible. Tannenbaum summarised this view in 1995: "Evidence-based medicine argues for the fundamental separability of expertise from expert and of knowledge from knower, and the distillation of medical truth outside the clinical encounter would seem to allow both buyers and sellers in the health care market to act independently and rationally."[6]

Although many disciples of the evidence based medicine movement (perhaps especially those with a management, rather than a clinical, background) might support this positivist image of evidence based practice, its founding fathers made no such claim for the objectivity of clinical method. Indeed, it was Sackett and his colleagues who found that whenever the diagnostic acumen of doctors is studied, different clinicians show a singularly unimpressive amount of agreement beyond chance.[7] Sackett et al argued that we should acknowledge and measure the amount of disagreement between different clinicians in different circumstances rather than dismiss it or attribute it to

Summary points

Even "evidence based" clinicians uphold the importance of clinical expertise and judgment

Clinical method is an interpretive act which draws on narrative skills to integrate the overlapping stories told by patients, clinicians, and test results

The art of selecting the most appropriate medical maxim for a particular clinical decision is acquired largely through the accumulation of "case expertise" (the stories or "illness scripts" of patients and clinical anecdotes)

The dissonance we experience when trying to apply research findings to the clinical encounter often occurs when we abandon the narrative-interpretive paradigm and try to get by on "evidence" alone

This is the last in a series of five articles on narrative based medicine

Department of Primary Care and Population Sciences, Royal Free and University College London Medical School, London N19 5NF
Trisha Greenhalgh, *senior lecturer*

p.greenhalgh@ucl.ac.uk

Series editor:
Trisha Greenhalgh

BMJ 1999;318:323–5

inexperience or incompetence. Clinical agreement, expressed statistically as the κ score, is of the order of 50% beyond chance for routine clinical procedures such as detecting the presence or absence of pulses in the feet, classifying diabetic retinopathy as mild or severe, and assessing the height of the jugular venous pressure. (Incidentally, cardiologists agreed rather more often than this in diagnosing angina from patients' descriptions of chest pain and, in some studies, rather less often in interpreting the abstracted, hard reality of electrocardiographic tracings.[7])

Those who have studied the phenomenon of clinical disagreement, as well as those of us who practise medicine in a clinical setting, know all too well that clinical judgments are usually a far cry from the objective analysis of a set of eminently measurable "facts." Pitting oedema, for example, will be more readily detected in a patient who has just mentioned that she ran out of "water tablets" last week than in someone who has made no such comment.

In the language of empiricism such an observation could be interpreted as ascertainment bias, but in the language of social constructionism it reflects the notion that even objective facts are theory laden.[8] Our medical training can be viewed as a kind of deductive narrative that predicts the fact of pitting oedema for which the trained clinical mind is then prepared. Evidence supports the claim that doctors do not simply assess symptoms and physical signs objectively: they interpret them by integrating the formal diagnostic criteria of the suspected disease (that is, what those diseases are supposed to do in "typical" patients as described in standard textbooks) with the case specific features of the patient's individual story and their own accumulated professional case expertise.

Originally published in *BMJ* 1999; **318**: 323–5.

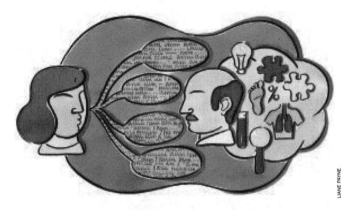

Diagnosis: evidence or the interpreted story?

We all know that anecdotal experience, the material of traditional medical practice and teaching,[9] is unrepresentative of the average case[10][11] and thus a potentially biased influence on decision making.[12] Evidence based clinical decision making involves the somewhat counterintuitive practice of assessing the current problem in the light of the aggregated results of hundreds or thousands of comparable cases in a distant population sample, expressed in the language of probability and risk—the stuff of clinical epidemiology[7] and bayesian statistics.[13]

How, then, can we square the circle of upholding individual narrative in a world where valid and generalisable truths come from population derived evidence? My own view is that there is no paradox. In particle physics the scientific truths (laws) derived from empirical observation about the behaviour of gases fail to hold when applied to single molecules. Similarly (but for different reasons), the "truths" established by the empirical observation of populations in randomised trials and cohort studies cannot be mechanistically applied to individual patients (whose behaviour is irremediably contextual and idiosyncratic) or episodes of illness.

In large research trials the individual participant's unique and multidimensional experience is expressed as (say) a single dot on a scatter plot to which we apply mathematical tools to produce a story about the sample as a whole. The generalisable truth that we seek to glean from research trials pertains to the sample's (and, hopefully, the population's) story, not the stories of individual participants. There is a serious danger of reifying that population story—that is, of applying what Whitehead called the fallacy of misplaced concreteness[14]—and erroneously viewing summary statistics as hard realities.

Misplaced concreteness is also an apt description of the dissonance we experience when we try to apply research evidence to clinical practice. Hunter has suggested that the reason why medical practice cannot constitute a science is that medicine lacks rules that can be generally and unconditionally applied to every case, even every case of a single disease.[15] This is borne out, for example, by Tudor Hart's observation that only 10% of patients in primary care have the sort of isolated, uncomplicated form of hypertension that lends itself to management by a standard evidence based guideline.[16] Hence, although there are certainly "wrong" answers to particular clinical questions, it is often impossible to define a single "right" one that can be applied in every context.

Integrated diagnostic judgments: evidence within the interpreted story

The box shows a comment made by a general practitioner in Cardiff, cited in a lecture by Nigel Stott, which I have expanded into a hypothetical example about Dr Jenkins. Meningococcal meningitis was diagnosed against the odds on the basis of two very non-specific symptoms and what was, on the face of it, a lucky hunch; the general practitioner who made the diagnosis had seen meningococcal meningitis only once in 96 000 consultations. Consider the decision sequence in this encounter: Dr Jenkins contemplates the brief history hastily obtained by the receptionist over the telephone and, using his intimate knowledge of the family, begins to put together the story of this illness.

One interpretation of this doctor's action is that he subconsciously compared the script so far with the tens of thousands of "illness scripts" from children over the years who had become (or were perceived to have become) acutely ill and decided that this script didn't fit with the template "nothing much the matter." The word "strangely" is rarely used by parents to describe the manifestations of non-specific illness in young children (compare the familiar expressions "off colour," "not herself," "poorly," "washed out," all of which occupy a very different semantic space from "strangely"[17]). It may be this single word that alerted the doctor to the seriousness of the case.

Of the many medical maxims (rules of thumb) that come to mind when trying to make sense of this story, Dr Jenkins might have taken particular note of the second and fifth maxims presented in the box to inform his decision making. This doctor's skill, which would be extremely difficult to measure formally, was to integrate judiciously selected best evidence (for example, on the prognosis of early meningococcal meningitis with and without the urgent administration of penicillin) with the potential significance of the word "strangely" and his personal knowledge about this family (their uncomplaining track record, the mother's

---

Dr Jenkins's hunch

"I got a call from a mother who said her little girl had had diarrhoea and was behaving strangely. I knew the family well, and was sufficiently concerned to break off my Monday morning surgery and visit immediately."

Maxims that might be considered in this case:

• We cannot commit ourselves completely and immediately to all patients who seek our help

• If meningococcal meningitis is suspected the doctor must act urgently and make the patient a priority

• Diarrhoea in previously well children is generally viral and self limiting

• Meningococcal meningitis produces a characteristic rash and neck stiffness

• Meningococcal meningitis presents non-specifically in primary care

good sense, and the memory of the child as one whose premorbid behaviour had been nothing out of the ordinary). Taken alone, neither best research evidence nor the intuitive response to a short but unusual story would have saved this patient, but the integrated application of both has produced a feat we would all be proud to replicate just once in our clinical careers.

The well documented frustration that health professionals experience when trying to apply evidence based research findings to real life case scenarios occurs most commonly when they abandon the interpretive framework and attempt to get by on evidence alone.[18-20] Such a situation might have occurred if Dr Jenkins had suspended his clinical judgment and adhered exclusively to the letter of a guideline on the early diagnosis and treatment of meningitis.

Stories within stories

The doctor-patient encounter takes place in a highly structured transactional space, in which the behaviour of both parties is determined by socialised expectations. In the American philosopher Leder's view, the "text" that constitutes the diagnostic encounter, and which distinguishes it from other human narratives or modes of communication, is a story about the "person as ill."[21] This in turn integrates four separate secondary texts:

● the experiential text—the meaning the patient assigns to the various symptoms, deliberations, and lay consultations in the run up to the clinical encounter (a subject eloquently explored by Heath[22]);

● the narrative text—what the doctor interprets to be "the problem" from the story the patient tells—the traditional medical history;

● the physical or perceptual text—what the doctor gleans from a physical examination of the patient (using the ill defined but recognisable set of skills that have been called "practical reason"[5]); and

● the instrumental text—what the blood tests and x rays "say."

In the instrumental text, "machines are employed to co-author a fuller story."[22] The shadow on the chest radiograph of a 19 year old student returning from an overland trip across India may be objectively identical to that of a 56 year old smoker who has never been out of Sweden. Both may have coughed up blood. But the radiologist who looks at the x ray films "sees" tuberculosis in one and a high probability of cancer in the other. According to Leder, the search for the "objective" analysis of diagnostic tests (for example, looking at an x ray film without a clinical or social history) is a flight from interpretation, and one that is doomed to fail.[21] This prediction from a hermeneutic perspective resonates strongly with the call from evidence based circles for the "truth" of the instrumental text (that is, the results of diagnostic tests) to be interpreted judiciously on the basis of bayesian pretest probabilities determined by the history and physical examination (for example, how likely on clinical grounds the patient is to have a particular condition).[7]

Leder's analysis and much of what has been written on the narrative stream in clinical medicine, centres on the diagnostic sequence, thus addressing only the first part of the clinical encounter. But there is also a therapeutic narrative: the formulation of a plan of what to do next and the enactment of that narrative.[23] Should the doctor order further tests, treat (if so, with what?), refer to a specialist colleague, or watch and wait? The increasing recognition that these decisions should arise out of informed dialogue between doctor and patient[24] has shown that there is a need for further research into the narrative of shared decision making[25]—an aspect of narrative analysis in medicine that will no doubt expand over the next few years.

Conclusion

Appreciating the narrative nature of illness experience and the intuitive and subjective aspects of clinical method does not require us to reject the principles of evidence based medicine. Nor does such an approach demand an inversion of the hierarchy of evidence so that personal anecdote carries more weight in decision making than the randomised controlled trial. Far from obviating the need for subjectivity in the clinical encounter, genuine evidence based practice actually presupposes an interpretive paradigm in which the patient experiences illness in a unique and contextual way. Furthermore, it is only within such an interpretive paradigm that a clinician can meaningfully draw on all aspects of evidence—his or her own case based experience, the patient's individual and cultural perspectives, and the results of rigorous clinical research trials and observational studies—to reach an integrated clinical judgment.

I thank the many colleagues who commented on earlier drafts of this article, in particular Dr Brian Hurwitz and Dr J A Muir Gray. The views expressed are mine alone.

1 Sackett DL, Rosenberg WMC, Gray JAM, Haynes RB, Richardson WS. Evidence based medicine: what it is and what it isn't. *BMJ* 1996;312:71-2.
2 Popper K. *Conjectures and refutations: the growth of scientific knowledge.* New York: Routledge and Kegan Paul, 1963.
3 McWhinney IR. Medical knowledge and the rise of technology. *J Med Philos* 1978;3:293-304.
4 Tannenbaum SJ. What physicians know. *N Engl J Med* 1993;329:1268-71.
5 Hunter KM. Narrative, literature, and the clinical exercise of practical reason. *J Med Philos* 1996;21:303-20.
6 Tannenbaum S. Getting there from here: evidentiary quandaries of the US outcomes movement. *J Eval Clin Pract* 1995;1:97-103.
7 Sackett DL, Haynes RB, Guyatt GH, Tugwell P. *Clinical epidemiology: a basic science for clinical medicine.* London: Little Brown, 1991.
8 Fish S. *Doing what comes naturally: change, rhetoric, and the practice of theory in literary and legal studies.* Durham, NC: Duke University Press, 1995.
9 Macnaughton J. Anecdote in clinical practice. In: Greenhalgh T, Hurwitz B, eds. *Narrative based medicine: dialogue and discourse in clinical practice.* London: BMJ Books, 1998:202-11.
10 Kahneman D, Slovic P, Tversky A. *Judgement under uncertainty: heuristics and biases.* Cambridge: Cambridge University Press, 1982.
11 Plous S. *The psychology of judgment and decision making.* New York: McGraw-Hill, 1993.
12 Dawson NV, Arkes HR. Systematic errors in medical decision making: judgement limitations. *Med Decis Making* 1987;2:183-7.
13 Freedman L. Bayesian statistical methods. *BMJ* 1996;313:569-70.
14 Whitehead AN. *Science and the modern world.* New York: Free Press, 1925.
15 Hunter K. "Don't think zebras": uncertainty, interpretation, and the place of paradox in clinical education. *Theor Med* 1996;17:225-41.
16 Tudor Hart JT. Hypertension guidelines: other diseases complicate management. *BMJ* 1993;306:1337.
17 Osgood C, May WH, Murray S. *Cross-cultural universals of affective meaning.* Urbana, IL: University of Illinois Press, 1975.
18 Grimley Evans J. Evidence-based and evidence biased medicine. *Age Ageing* 1995;25:461-4.
19 Asch DA. Why some health policies don't make sense at the bedside. *Ann Intern Med* 1995;122:846-50.
20 Greenhalgh T. Evidence-based medicine. In: Hall M, Dwyer D, Lewis T, eds. *GP training handbook.* 3rd ed. Oxford: Blackwell Scientific, 1998.
21 Leder D. Clinical interpretation: the hermeneutics of medicine. *Theor Med* 1990;11:9-24.
22 Heath I. *The mystery of general practice.* London: Nuffield Provincial Hospitals Trust, 1995:17-21.
23 Mattingly C. The concept of therapeutic emplotment. *Soc Sci Med* 1994;34:811-22.
24 Stewart M. *Patient centred medicine.* London: Sage, 1995.
25 Elwyn GJ. *Shared decision making in primary care.* Cardiff: Welsh Office, 1997.

UNIT 3 *Approaching the literature*

SUGGESTED AIM FOR THIS SESSION

To allow participants to become confident in approaching electronic clinical databases with focused and potentially answerable clinical questions.

SUGGESTED LEARNING OBJECTIVES FOR THIS SESSION

By the end of this session, participants will be able to:
- distinguish questions that can potentially be answered from the research literature from those that require other sources of information;
- derive and prioritise focused and answerable questions from an undifferentiated clinical problem;
- identify appropriate research designs (for example, randomised controlled trial, cohort study) for each question;
- construct and modify a search strategy to retrieve high-quality, relevant research articles;
- refine the search if necessary if too many or too few articles are identified.

SET ARTICLES

1. Greenhalgh T. How to read a paper. The Medline database. *BMJ* 1997; **315**: 180–3. [A longer version of this article appears in Greenhalgh T. *How to read a paper: the basics of evidence-based medicine.* London: BMJ Books, 1997. See in particular Chapter 2: Searching the literature, pages 13–33.
2. Glanville J, Haines M, Auston I. Finding information on clinical effectiveness. *BMJ* 1998; **317**: 200–3.

THE FOUR-PART CLINICAL QUESTION

Scott Richardson and Dave Sackett produced an elegant and widely applicable framework for generating the kind of question that will enable you to retrieve high-quality and relevant material from the clinical literature (see Further Reading for references). The sequence is as follows:
1. List all the main questions arising from your clinical problem.
2. Select those that are potentially answerable from information in the research literature (as opposed to, for example, the clinical case notes, the patient's values and preferences or details of local health care services).
3. Use the acronym PICO (Population–Intervention–Comparison–Outcome) for therapy questions and PEO (Population–Exposure–Outcome) to construct a focused clinical question as illustrated below.

Element	Suggestions to help	Example
1. The patient or population	"How would I succinctly describe a group of patients similar to this one?"	In children under 12 years with poorly controlled asthma on medium-dose inhaled steroids ...
2. The intervention (test, treatment, risk factor) being considered	"What is the main action I am considering?"	... would adding salmeterol to their current therapy ...
3. The comparison or alternative (where relevant)	"What is (are) the other option(s)?"	... compared to increasing the dose of their current therapy ...
4. The outcome(s) of interest	"What do/es I/the patient want to happen/not happen?"	... lead to increased symptom control with no increase in side effects?

SUGGESTIONS FOR GROUP EXERCISE

Invite members of the group to share case histories of clinical encounters they have experienced, either as health professionals or as patients or carers. Have a "brainstorming" session with a flip chart to generate a range of questions around one of these cases. Classify each question in terms of the information source needed to answer it: "clinical casenotes", "facts from patient", "values/preferences from patient", "research literature", "resources", "local services", "unanswerable", and so on. You will probably find that some questions need breaking down into several more specific questions before they can be classified.

What proportion of questions appear answerable from the research literature? If you are a multidisciplinary group, identify which professional group asked the most research-oriented questions and which the least. Who asked the most questions about the patient's experience and about other aspects of the problem?

Sample case history for generating clinical questions

A 25-year-old Pakistani woman, newly immigrated to the UK, presents to her GP. Her husband is a lawyer and they both speak perfect English. She is 30 weeks pregnant. She says she has recently been told by a doctor in Pakistan that she is "mildly thalassaemic". She is taking oral iron.

On examination she is small (150 cm), underweight (42 kg), and pale. The size of the abdominal swelling is consistent with her dates and there is no other physical abnormality. The GP finds glucose ++ in the urine and asks her to go for a blood test. The patient agrees but fails to attend.

SUGGESTIONS FOR INDIVIDUAL STUDY

1. Try the exercise based on the case history above.
2. During a clinical encounter (if you are a clinician) or during a meeting or seminar in which aspects of public health or health policy are being discussed (if you are an epidemiologist or a manager), note down a list of questions that come to you about the topic

under discussion. Afterwards, classify the questions as described above and reflect on the most likely source of answers for each category.

FURTHER READING

Adams CE, Lefebre C, Chalmers I. Difficulties with MEDLINE searches for randomised controlled trials. *Lancet* 1992; **340**: 915–16.

Armstrong EC. The well-built clinical question: the key to finding the best evidence efficiently. *Western Med J* 1999; **98**: 25–8.

Haynes RB, Johnston ME, McKibbon KA, Walker CJ, Willan AR. A program to enhance clinical use of MEDLINE. A randomized controlled trial. *Online J Curr Clin Trials* 1993.

Jadad AR, Haynes RB. The Cochrane collaboration – advances and challenges in improving evidence-based decision making. *Med Decis Making* 1998; **18**: 2–9.

Kim P, Eng TR, Deering MJ, Maxfield A. Published criteria for evaluating health related web sites: review. *BMJ* 1999; **318**: 96–100.

Sackett D, Richardson WS, Rosenberg W, Haynes RB. *Evidence-based medicine: how to practise and teach EBM.* London: Churchill Livingstone, 1997. See in particular Chapter 1: How to ask clinical questions you can answer, pages 21–36.

How to read a paper: The Medline database

Trisha Greenhalgh, *senior lecturer* [a]

[a] Unit for Evidence-Based Practice and Policy, Department of PrimaryCare and Population Sciences, University College London Medical School/Royal Free Hospital School of Medicine, Whittington Hospital, London N19 5NF, p.greenhalgh@ucl.ac.uk

 ## Introduction

In 1928, in his introduction to *Sceptical Essays*, Bertrand Russell wrote: "The extent to which beliefs are based on evidence is very much less than believers suppose." Medical beliefs, and the clinical practices that are based on them, are a case in point. Debate continues as to whether scientific evidence alone is sufficient to guide medical decision making, but few doctors would dispute that finding and understanding relevant research based evidence is increasingly necessary in clinical practice. This article is the first in a series that introduces the non-expert to searching the medical literature and assessing the value of medical articles.

 ## The Medline database

Over 10 million medical articles exist on library shelves. About a third are indexed in the huge Medline database, compiled by the National Library of Medicine of the United States. The Medline database is exactly the same, whichever company is selling it, but the commands differ according to the software. Vendors of Medline online and on CD ROM include Ovid Technologies (ovid) and Silver Platter Information (WinSPIRS).

Articles can be traced in two ways: by any word listed on the database, including words in the title, abstract, authors' names, and the institution where the research was done; and by a restricted thesaurus of medical titles, known as medical subject heading (MeSH) terms.

To illustrate how Medline works, I have worked through some common problems in searching. The scenarios have been drawn up using ovid software.

Problem 1: You are trying to find a known paper
Solution: Search the database by field suffix (title, author, journal, institution, etc) or by textwords.

First, get into the part of the database which covers the approximate year of the paper's publication. If you are already in the main Medline menu, select "database" (Alt-B). If you know the approximate title of the paper and perhaps the journal where it was published, you can use the title and journal search keys or (this is quicker) the **.ti** and **.jn** field suffixes. The box shows some other useful field suffixes.

Originally published in *BMJ* Education and debate 1998, **315**: 180–3.

Useful search field suffixes (ovid)		
Syntax	**Meaning**	**Example**
.ab	Word in abstract	**epilepsy.ab**
.au	Author	**smith-r.au**
.jn	Journal	**lancet.jn**
.me	Single word, wherever it may appear as a MeSH term	**ulcer.me**
.ti	Word in title	**epilepy.ti**
.tw	Word in title or abstract	**epilepsy.tw**
.ui	Unique identifier	**91574637.ui**
.yr	Year of publication	**87.yr**

Thus, to find a paper called something like "Confidentiality and patients' casenotes", which you remember seeing in the *British Journal of General Practice* a couple of years ago,[1] type the following sequence:

1. confidentiality.ti

2. british journal of general practice.jn

3. 1 and 2

Summary points

Not all medical articles are indexed on Medline, and many that are have been misclassified

Searching by textword can supplement a search by MeSH headings

To increase the sensitivity of a search, use the "explode" command and avoid using subheadings

Scan titles on screen rather than relying on the software to find the most valid or relevant ones

You could do all this in one step:

1. confidentiality.ti and british journal of general practice.jn

This step illustrates the use of the boolean operator "and"; it will give you articles common to both sets. Using "or" will simply add the two sets together.

Note that since 1988 the *British Medical Journal* is abbreviated BMJ in ovid software, and *Journal of the American Medical Association* is JAMA. Other useful field suffixes to try when searching for a known article are author (using the syntax haines-ap.au), institution (for example, manchester.in), or title (for example, evidence-based medicine.ti).

Problem 2: You want to answer a specific question
Solution: Construct a focused (specific) search by combining two or more broad (sensitive) searches.

I was recently asked by the mother of a young girl with anorexia nervosa whose periods had ceased to prescribe oral contraceptives for her so as to stop her bones thinning. This seemed a reasonable request, though there were ethical problems to consider. But is there any evidence that taking oral contraceptives in these circumstances really prevents long term bone loss? I decided to explore the subject using Medline. To answer this question, you need to search very broadly under "anorexia nervosa," "osteoporosis," and "oral contraceptives." The search described below involves articles from 1992; when replicating it, make sure the database you are searching goes back that far. Type:

1 anorexia nervosa

You have not typed a field suffix (such as .tw), so the ovid system will automatically try to "map" your request to one of its standard medical subject headings (abbreviated MeSH and colloquially known as "mesh terms"). (Note that not all Medline software packages will automatically map your suggestion to MeSH terms. With Silver Platter search software, for example, you need to enter your heading and click the "suggest" button.) For this example, the screen offers you either "eating disorders" or "anorexia nervosa" and asks you to pick the closest one. Choose "anorexia nervosa" (space bar to highlight the text, then press "return"). The screen then asks you whether you want to "restrict to focus." Do you only want articles which are actually about anorexia nervosa in passing? Let's say we do want to restrict to focus. Next, the screen offers us a choice of subheadings, but we'll ignore these for a moment. Select "Include all subheadings." We could have got this far using a single line command:

2 *anorexia nervosa/

The * shows that the term is a major focus of the article, and the / represents a MeSH term. You should have about 750 articles in this set.

Similarly, to get articles on osteoporosis (which is also a MeSH term), use the following single line command:

3 osteoporosis/

You should get about 2200 articles. Note that in ovid, if you know that the subject you want is an official MeSH term, you can shortcut the mapping process by typing a slash (/) after the word. Note also that we have not used an asterisk here, because osteoporosis may not be the focus of the article we are looking for.

Finally, put in the term "oral contraceptives" (without an asterisk and without a slash) to see what the MeSH term here is. You will be offered "contraceptives, oral," and if you had known this you could have used the following command:

4 contraceptives, oral/

This set should contain around 1200 articles. You can combine these three sets, either by using their set numbers 1 and 2 and 3 or by typing the single line command:

5 *anorexia nervosa/ and osteoporosis/ and contraceptives, oral/

With this you will have searched over 4000 articles and struck a single bull's eye.[2] (If you don't find it, check the syntax of your search carefully, then try running the same search through the previous five year database using the Alt-B command.)

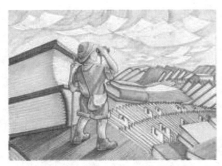

Problem 3: You want to get general information quickly about a well defined topic
Solution: Use subheadings and/or the "limit set" options.

Subheadings are the fine tuning of the Medline indexing system; they classify articles on a particular MeSH topic into aetiology, prevention, therapy, and so on. The most useful ones are listed in the box. I try not to use subheadings unless I have unearthed an unmanageable set of articles, since an estimated 50% of articles in Medline are inadequately or incorrectly classified by subheading. It actually doesn't take long to browse through 50 or so articles on the screen. It is better to do this than to rely on the "limit set" command (see box) to give you the best of the bunch.

Useful subheadings (ovid)

Syntax	Meaning	Example
/ae	Adverse effects	thalidomide/ae
/co	Complications	measles/co
/ct	Contraindications (of drug)	propranolol/ct
/di	Diagnosis	glioma/di
/dt	Drug therapy	depression/dt
/ed	Education	asthma/ed
/ep	Epidemiology	poliomyelitis/ep
/hi	History	mastectomy/hi
/nu	Nursing	cerebral palsy/nu
/og	Organisation/administration	health service/og
/pc	Prevention and control	influenza/pc
/px	Psychology	diabetes/px
/th	Therapy	hypertension/th
/tu	Therapeutic use (of drug)	aspirin/tu

Useful "limit set" options	
AIM journals	Abstracts
Nursing journals	Local holdings
Dental journals	English language
Cancer journals	Male
Review articles	Human
Editorials	Publication year

The option "AIM journals" denotes all journals listed in the Abridged Index Medicus—that is, the "mainstream" medical journals. Alternatively, if you want articles relating to nursing, rather than medical care, you could limit the set to "Nursing journals." This is often a better way of limiting a large set than asking for local holdings. If you are not interested in seeing anything in a foreign language (even though the abstract may be in English), select this option, again bearing in mind that it is a non-systematic (indeed, a very biased) way of excluding articles from your set.[3]

Note that instead of using the "limit set" function key you can use direct single line commands such as:

9 limit 4 to local holdings

10 limit 5 to human

Problem 4: Your search gives irrelevant articles
Solution: Refine your search as you go along in the light of interim results.

Often, a search uncovers dozens of articles which are irrelevant to your question. The boolean operator "not" can help here. I recently undertook a search to identify articles on surrogate endpoints in clinical pharmacology research. My search revealed hundreds of articles I didn't want—all on surrogate motherhood. The syntax to exclude the unwanted articles is:

1 (surrogate not mother$).tw

Deciding to use the "not" operator is a good example of how you can (and should) refine your search as you go along—much easier than producing the perfect search off the top of your head. I used the truncation symbol **$** to find all words from a single stem, such as mother, mothers, motherhood, and so on.

Another way of getting rid of irrelevant articles is to narrow your textword search to adjacent words using the "adj" operator. For example, the term "home help" includes two very common words linked in a specific context. Link them as follows:

1 home adj help.tw

Problem 5: The search gives no articles, or too few
Solution: Firstly, don't overuse subheadings or the "limit set" options. Secondly, search under textwords as well as MeSH terms. Thirdly, learn about the "explode" command, and use it routinely.

Many important articles are missed not because we constructed a flawed search strategy but because we relied too heavily on a flawed indexing system. For this reason, you should adopt a "belt and braces" approach and search under textwords as well as by MeSH terms. After all, it is difficult to write an article on the psychology of diabetes without mentioning the words "diabetes," "diabetic," "psychology," or "psychological," so the truncation stems "diabet$.tw." and "psychol$.tw." would supplement a search under the MeSH term "diabetes mellitus" and the subheading "/px" (psychology).

Another important strategy for preventing incomplete searches is to use the powerful "explode" command. The MeSH terms are like the branches of a tree with, for example, "asthma" subdividing into "asthma in children," "occupational asthma," and so on. Medline indexers are instructed to index items by using the most specific MeSH terms they can. If you just ask for articles on "asthma" you will miss all the articles indexed under "asthma in children" unless you "explode" the term using the following syntax:

1 exp asthma/

Problem 6: You don't know where to start searching
Solution: Use the "permuted index" option.

Let's take the term "stress." It comes up often, but searching for particular types of stress would be laborious and searching "stress" as a textword would be too unfocused. We need to know where in the MeSH index the various types of stress lie, and when we see that, we can choose the sort of stress we want to look at. For this, we use the command ptx ("permuted index"):

1 ptx stress

The screen shows many options, including post-traumatic stress disorders, stress fracture, oxidative stress, stress incontinence, and so on.

The command "ptx" is useful when the term might be found in several subject areas. If your subject is a discrete MeSH term, use the tree command. For example:

2 tree epilepsy

will show where epilepsy is placed in the MeSH index—as a branch of "brain diseases," which itself branches into generalised epilepsy, partial epilepsy, post-traumatic epilepsy, and so on.

Problem 7: Limiting a set loses important articles but does not exclude those of low methodological quality
Solution: Apply an EBQF (evidence based quality filter).

If your closely focused search still gives you several hundred articles, and if applying subheadings or limit set functions seems to lose valuable (and valid) papers, you should insert a quality string designed to limit your set to therapeutic interventions, aetiology, diagnostic procedures, or epidemiology. Alternatively, you could apply search strings to identify the publication type, such as randomised controlled trial, systematic review, or meta-analysis.

These EBQFs (evidence based quality filters), which are listed in Appendix 1, are complex search strategies developed by some of the world's most experienced medical information experts. You can copy them into your personal computer and save them as strategies to be added to your subject searches. Other search strategies that will identify cohort studies, case-control studies, and so on will soon be available from the UK Cochrane Centre, Summertown Pavillion, Middle Way, Oxford OX2 7LG (general@cochrane.co.uk).

Problem 8: Medline hasn't helped
Solution: Explore other medical and paramedical databases .

Entry of articles onto the Medline database is open to human error, both from authors and editors who select key words for indexing, and from the librarians who group articles under subheadings and type in the abstracts. In addition, some sections of indexed journals are not available on Medline (for example, the News section of the *BMJ*). According to one estimate, 40% of material which should be listed on Medline can, in reality, only be accessed by looking through all the journals again, by hand. Furthermore, a number of important medical and paramedical journals are not covered by Medline at all. It is said that Medline lacks comprehensive references in the fields of psychology, medical sociology, and non-clinical pharmacology.

If you wish to broaden your search to other electronic databases, ask your local librarian where you could access the following:

- *AIDSLINE* — Covers AIDS and HIV back to 1980.

- *Allied and Alternative Medicine* — Covers complementary and alternative medicine.

- *American Medical Association Journals* — Provides the full text of JAMA plus 10 specialty journals produced by the American Medical Association; from 1982.

- *ASSIA* — An applied social sciences database covering psychology, sociology, politics, and economics since 1987. All documents have abstracts.

- *Cancer-CD* — A compilation by Silver Platter of cancerlit and Embase cancer related records from 1984. The CD ROM version is updated quarterly.

- *CINAHL* — The nursing and allied health database covering all aspects of nursing, health education, occupational therapy, social services in health care, and other related disciplines from 1983. The CD ROM version is updated monthly.

- *Cochrane Library* — The Cochrane Controlled Trials Register (cctr), Cochrane Database of Systematic Reviews (cdsr), Database of Abstracts of Reviews of Effectiveness (dare), and Cochrane Review Methodology Database (crmd) are updated quarterly; authors of systematic reviews on cdsr undertake to update their own contributions periodically.[4]

- *Current Contents Search* — Indexes journal issues on or before their publication date. It is useful when checking for the very latest output on a subject. Updated weekly; from 1990.

- *Current Research in Britain* — The British national research database of trials in progress.

- *DHData* (formerly DHSS-Data) — The database of the UK's Department of Health indexes articles covering health service and hospital administration; from 1983.

- *Embase* — Focuses on drugs and pharmacology but also includes other biomedical specialties. It is more up to date than Medline and has better European coverage. The CD ROM version is updated monthly.

- *HELMIS* — The Health Management Information Service at the Nuffield Institute of Health, Leeds, UK, indexes articles on health service management.

- *Psychlit* — Produced by the American Psychological Association as the computer searchable version of Psychological Abstracts; covers psychology, psychiatry, and related subjects; journals are included from 1974 and books from 1987 (English language only).

- *Science Citation Index* — Indexes references cited in articles as well as the usual author, title, abstract, and citation of articles themselves. Useful for finding follow up work done on a key article and for tracking down addresses of authors.

- *SHARE* — Based at the King's Fund library in London; published and ongoing research into the health of, and health services for, black and minority ethnic groups.

- *Toxline* — Information on toxicological effects of chemicals and drugs on living systems; from 1981.

- *UNICORN* — The main database of the King's Fund, London. Covers health, health management, health economics, and social sciences. Particularly strong on primary health care and the health of Londoners.

▶ Acknowledgements

Thanks to Mr Reinhard Wentz, Ms Jane Rowlands, Ms Carol Lefebvre, and Ms Valerie Wildridge for advice on this chapter. I am grateful to Carol Lefebvre of the UK Cochrane Centre for permission to reproduce the EBQFs in Appendix 1.

▶ References

1. Caman D, Britten N. Confidentiality and medical records: the patient's perspective. *Br J Gen Prac* 1995;**45**:485–8.
2. Seeman E, Szmukler GI, Formica C, Tsalamandris C, Mestrovic R. Osteoporosis in anorexia nervosa: the influence of peak bone density, bone loss, oral contraceptive use, and exercise. *J Bone Mineral Res* 1992;**7**:1467–74.
3. Moher D, Fortin P, Jadad AR, Juni P, Klassen T, Le Lorier J, et al. Completeness of reporting of trials published in languages other than English: implications for conduct and reporting of systematic reviews. *Lancet* 1996;**347**:363–6.
4. Bero L, Rennie D. The Cochrane Collaboration: preparing, maintaining, and disseminating systematic reviews of the effects of health care. *JAMA* 1995;**274**:1935–8.

Appendix 1: Evidence based quality filters for everyday use

(a) Therapeutic interventions (What works?)

1. exp clinical trials

2. exp research design

3. randomized controlled trial.pt.

4. clinical trial.pt.

5. (single or double or treble or triple).tw.

6. (mask$ or blind$).tw.

7. 5 and 6

8. placebos/ or placebo.tw.

9. 1 or 2 or 3 or 4 or 7 or 8

(b) Aetiology (What causes it? What are the risk factors?)

1. exp causality

2. exp cohort studies

3. exp risk

4. 1 or 2 or 3

(c) Diagnostic procedures

1. exp "sensitivity and specificity"

2. exp diagnostic errors

3. exp mass screening

4. 1 or 2 or 3

(d) Epidemiology

1. sn.xs

(This would find all articles indexed under any MeSH term with any of "statistics," "epidemiology," "ethnology," or "mortality" as subheadings.)

Appendix 2: Maximally sensitive search strings (to be used mainly for research)

(a) Maximally sensitive qualifying string for randomised controlled trials

1. RANDOMIZED CONTROLLED TRIAL.pt.

2. CONTROLLED CLINICAL TRIAL.pt.

3. RANDOMIZED CONTROLLED TRIALS.sh.

4. RANDOM ALLOCATION .sh.

5. DOUBLE–BLIND METHOD.sh.

6. SINGLE–BLIND METHOD.sh.

7. or/1-6

8. ANIMAL.sh. not HUMAN.sh.

9. 7 not 8

10. CLINICAL TRIAL.pt.

11. exp CLINICAL TRIALS

12. (clin$ adj25 trial$).ti,ab.

13. ((single or double or treble or triple) adj25 (blind$ or mas$)).ti,ab.

14. PLACEBOS.sh.

15. placebo$.ti,ab.

16. random$.ti,ab.

17. RESEARCH DESIGN.sh.

18. or/10-17

19. 18 not 8

20. 19 not 9

21. COMPARATIVE STUDY .sh.

22. exp EVALUATION STUDIES /

23. FOLLOW UP STUDIES.sh.

24. PROSPECTIVE STUDIES.sh.

25. (control$ or prospectiv$ or volunteer$).ti,ab.

26. or/21-25

27. 26 not 8

28. 26 not (9 or 20)

29. 9 or 20 or 28

In these examples, upper case denotes controlled vocabulary and lower case denotes free text terms. Search statements 8, 9, 19, and 27 could be omitted if your search takes too long a time to run.

(b) Maximally sensitive qualifying string for identifying systematic reviews

1. REVIEW, ACADEMIC .pt.

2. REVIEW, TUTORIAL .pt.

3. META–ANALYSIS .pt.

4. META–ANALYSIS .sh.

5. systematic$ adj25 review$

6. systematic$ adj25 overview$

7. meta-analy$ or metaanaly$ or (meta analy$)

8. or/1-7

9. ANIMAL.sh. not HUMAN.sh.

10. 8 not 9

Search statements 9 and 10 could be omitted if your search seems to be taking a long time to run.

Getting research findings into practice

Finding information on clinical effectiveness

This is the third in a series of eight articles analysing the gap between research and practice

Julie Glanville, *information service manager,*[a] **Margaret Haines,** *principal adviser,*[b]
Ione Auston, *librarian.*[c]

[a] NHS Centre for Reviews and Dissemination,
University of York, York Y01 5DD, [b] Library and Information Commission, London W1V 4BH, [c] National Information
Center on Health Services Research and Health Care Technology, National Library of Medicine, 8600 Rockville Pike,
Bethesda, MD 20894, USA

Correspondence to: Ms Glanville

Series editors: Andrew Haines and Anna Donald

There is increasing pressure on healthcare professionals to ensure that their practice is based on
evidence from good quality research, such as randomised controlled trials or, preferably, systematic
reviews of randomised controlled trials and trials of other study designs. This pressure comes from
various sources. The evidence based healthcare movement encourages a questioning and reflective
approach to clinical practice and emphasises the importance of lifelong learning. Thus, good access to
research based evidence is necessary. Many governments are encouraging the development of
evidence based medicine because its advantages are understood, especially in terms of improved
efficiency in the delivery of health care through the identification of effective treatments. [1] [2] There are
also indications that legal decisions may take account of whether research evidence and clinical
guidelines were adhered to. [3] [4] Better informed consumers may provide another incentive for
clinicians to be more aware of research findings. Clinicians will need to be able to access information
on clinical effectiveness in order to improve the quality of care and to stay well informed on
developments in specialist areas. We examine the resources that are already available to clinicians,
strategies for finding and filtering information, and ways of improving dissemination.

Originally published in *BMJ* 1998; **317**: 200–203.

Summary points

Information alone is often not sufficient to encourage changes in practice

A national dissemination strategy for important research messages combined with local support mechanisms may increase the uptake of changes in practice

All healthcare decision makers need to know how to filter research for quality and how to appraise evidence from research

Extensive information on clinical effectiveness is already available, and computer based systems are being developed that will present clinicians with evidence based information when they need it

Good library and information support provided to doctors has been proved to make a positive impact on clinical decision making

Evidence based information already available

In the 1990s evidence from research has become more easily available. In part this has been due to the development of programmes for assessing health technology and to the growth in systematic reviews. Systematic reviews evaluate primary evidence and the effectiveness of particular interventions. They necessarily take time to complete but a useful compilation of reviews is available in *The Cochrane Library* and there are also reports from technology assessment agencies such as the Agency for Health Care Policy and Research in the United States or in England the Department of Health's health technology assessment programme. The publications and databases in the box present evidence on effectiveness, often in a summarised form suitable for the busy clinician or policymaker. However, important problems remain, such as how to increase awareness of what information is available and how to provide clinicians with information when they need it.

Selected resources

The Cochrane Library

A collection of databases including the full text of the *Cochrane Database of Systematic Reviews*, critical commentaries on selected systematic reviews that have been assessed for quality by the NHS Centre for Reviews and Dissemination, and brief details of more than 170 000 randomised controlled trials.

Available from : Update Software, Summertown Pavilion, Middle Way, Summertown, Oxford, OX2 7LG, or http://www.medlib.com and http://www.hcn.net.au/

Clinical Guidelines from the US Agency for Health Care Policy and Research

A series of clinical guidelines based on thorough reviews of research evidence. The agency is now focusing on producing evidence reports (reviews and analyses of scientific literature designed to provide the basis for guidelines, measures of performance, and other tools for quality improvement), as well as working with the American Medical Association and the American Association of Health Plans to develop an online clearing house for practice guidelines; the online service will have electronic mailing lists to keep users informed about the implementation of guidelines.

Available from : http://text.nlm.nih.gov/ and http://www.ahcpr.gov:80/news/press/ngc.html

Best Evidence Database on CD ROM

Abstracts of primary and review articles that have been published in the *American College of Physicians Journal Club* and *Evidence-Based Medicine* , with assessments of quality by clinical experts.

Available from : BMJ Publishing, London WC1H 9JR, or http://hiru.hirunet.mcmaster.ca/acpjc

Effective Health Care Bulletins

Reports of systematic reviews presented in a readable and accessible format, produced by the NHS Centre for Reviews and Dissemination.

Available from : Subscriptions Department, Pearson Professional, PO Box 77, Fourth Avenue, Harlow CM19 5BQ, or http://www.york.ac.uk/inst/crd

Guide to Clinical Preventive Services, 2nd ed

US Preventive Services Task Force. Baltimore: Williams and Wilkins, 1996

Evidence based recommendations on preventive services.

Available from : http://text.nlm.nih.gov/

Canadian Guide to Clinical Preventive Health Care

Ottawa: Health Canada, 1994

Evidence based recommendations on preventive services.

Bandolier

UK newsletter alerting readers to key evidence about effectiveness in health care.

Available from : http://www.jr2.ox.ac.uk/Bandolier

Drug and Therapeutics Bulletin

Independent assessments of drugs and other treatments.

Available from : Consumers' Association, Castlemead, Gascoyne Way, Hertford, SG14 1LH

Effectiveness Matters

Summaries of published research on a single topic which emphasise presenting clear messages on effectiveness.

Available from : NHS Centre for Reviews and Dissemination, University of York, York Y01 5DD, or http://www.york.ac.uk/inst/crd

> **MeReC Bulletin**
>
> Reviews of new drugs compiled for general practitioners, with discussion of effectiveness, safety, appropriateness, acceptability, and cost.
>
> *Available from* : Medicines Resource Centre, Hamilton House, 24 Pall Mall, Liverpool L3 6AL
>
> **NHS Economic Evaluation Database**
>
> Critical assessments of published economic evaluations, produced by the NHS Centre for Reviews and Dissemination.
>
> *Available from* : NHS Centre for Reviews and Dissemination, University of York, York Y01 5DD, or http://nhscrd.york.ac.uk/Welcome.html

Collections of systematic reviews and critical appraisals of primary research are valuable sources of evaluated research. The proliferation of these collections is creating its own information explosion; this is a serious problem that needs to be addressed. Because there is no single comprehensive index to all the material described in the box several searches through both paper journals and electronic services may be required to locate relevant information. It may also be necessary to obtain copies of the original publication. These are disincentives to searching for and obtaining research evidence. Information technology may eventually provide a more streamlined way of dealing with this explosion of information, perhaps in the form of world wide web interfaces that provide links to a range of evidence based information services that filter publications for quality, or by providing access to the full text of publications. Biomednet is one model of this type of service. It offers a range of full text resources with free Medline access, discussion facilities, and virtual meeting rooms. Biomednet is beginning to highlight important papers that have been cited and evaluated by expert reviewers as a means of filtering papers for quality.[5]

The resources in the box provide information that has been evaluated and filtered–that is, they highlight the best quality studies from the mass of available literature. However, research based answers to many questions of effectiveness are not yet available in such time saving, value added forms. Clinicians may still need to search indexes and abstracts of published literature. For several years it has been possible for clinicians to search Medline using software such as Grateful Med, and its world wide web interface, internet Grateful Med. This has provided access to a large body of peer reviewed studies that are mostly unsynthesised and unevaluated. There are tools to help searchers identify the types of studies that are more likely to provide high quality information on clinical effectiveness, such as systematic reviews or randomised controlled trials.[6 7] Once the original papers have been retrieved there are checklists that, together with training in critical appraisal skills, can be used to assess the rigour and validity of such studies.[8-10]

Although Medline is a rich resource, access is increasingly required to a wider range of material than it presently indexes. The US National Library of Medicine and the American Hospital Association have recently launched the HealthSTAR database which seeks to provide expanded access to both non-clinical information (on topics such as healthcare administration, economics, and planning) and non-journal information (such as reports, meeting abstracts, and chapters from books) that is not available in journals.[11] The National Library of Medicine has recently announced that access to Medline and HealthSTAR through internet Grateful Med and access to Medline through the PubMed interface will be free.[11] Other databases that cover specific clinical areas, specific types of publications, and non-English language material should also be used. Tools such as search strategies and single interfaces, like PubMed, are required to enhance access to a range of such databases.

 ## Strategies for finding and filtering information

Training and practice are required to search information services and navigate the internet effectively, but other options are available which may help clinicians cope with the challenges of finding information. Locating, appraising, and exploiting resources, both print and electronic, has typically been the role of the librarian or information professional. Increasingly, clinicians are finding that librarians can not only help them locate information in answer to a particular question but also can help to keep their knowledge up to date by presenting selections of important new evidence in the form of paper or electronic bulletins.

The value of library and information support has been demonstrated on both sides of the Atlantic. Trained librarians are often more effective than physicians in filtering papers for quality.[12] Some American studies have shown that library support not only contributes to lower patient care costs by decreasing the number of admissions, length of stay, and number of procedures but also contributes to a higher quality of care in terms of patient advice, improved decision making, and savings in time. [13] [14] A similar study in the United Kingdom found that library services had a positive impact on the continuing education of hospital doctors.[15]

Not all clinicians have the time to visit libraries, and new models have emerged for delivering library support directly to hospital wards and departments. [16] [17] In the United States, the National Network of Libraries of Medicine provides outreach services to general practitioners (and, more recently, to public health professionals); in the United Kingdom the BMA library offers an electronic outreach service to members. [18] [19] Also in the United Kingdom, the Oxford PRISE (primary care sharing the evidence) project is developing a model whereby general practitioners' computers are linked to a central computer that provides access to a range of databases; in this model the general practitioners can also request librarians to follow up particular questions in more detail.[20] Librarians are increasingly asked to provide training in information skills as part of courses in evidence based medicine offered to NHS staff.

The development of primary care based services presents a challenge to librarians; they must become better trained to deal with a wider range of inquiries, to evaluate and synthesise evidence, and to present selected information through innovative delivery systems. Clearly initiatives such as the Oxford Health Libraries' training programme, known as the "librarian of the 21st century," is a model for other library networks.[21] Similar initiatives under development in the United States include the National Information Center on Health Services Research and Health Care Technology, web based training materials that are not copyrighted and can be modified to suit the user,[22] and training programmes for librarians sponsored by the National Library of Medicine in subjects such as medical informatics.

Improving dissemination

For information to be accessible it must be packaged and published in formats that promote easy identification and encourage use. Evidence based information is becoming easier to find: structured abstracts in articles in journals make it easier to identify the methodology of a study and its potential reliability. Innovations, such as the *BMJ*'s key messages boxes, make it easier to identify the important points of research. Journal editors have an important role in encouraging authors to provide informative abstracts and in ensuring that researchers' conclusions are supported by their paper's results. However, the benefits of clearer labelling may be undermined if current buzz words, such as

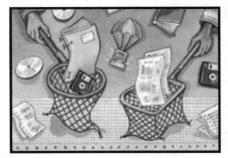

"effective" and "evidence based", are adopted and used incorrectly or inaccurately so that previously useful labels become meaningless.

Organisations that produce recommendations on policy and clinical guidelines are finding it necessary to make their guidelines more explicitly evidence based, both by using research evidence to develop their guidelines and in stating the level of evidence on which the guidance is based. [23] [24] It would be easier and quicker to assess guidelines if the types of evidence used in their development were stated as clearly as possible, for example on the front cover of published guidelines there could be a statement to the effect that "this guideline is based on a Cochrane review." The guideline appraisal project of the Health Information Research Unit at McMaster University is an example of efforts to help practitioners identify and critically evaluate clinical guidelines, and to determine their applicability to local practice.[25]

Information from research needs to be presented in forms that are appropriate for the target audience. Guidelines from the Agency for Health Care Policy and Research have been packaged in different ways for different users; they have been packaged as a detailed report of the review with a full exposition of the evidence for researchers and decision makers, as a briefer guideline for clinicians, and as a leaflet for patients. In the United Kingdom, the Midwives Information and Resource Service has produced a series of leaflets aimed at both pregnant women and their professional carers using, when possible, evidence from Cochrane reviews.[26]

Simply presenting research evidence to clinicians is often insufficient to ensure that it is incorporated into practice. Government directives and direct incentives such as payments can increase the speed of uptake. Sometimes powerful research findings will have an immediate effect; swift changes in practice followed the publication of research findings that sleeping position could affect mortality from the sudden infant death syndrome. [27] [28] However, even when findings are packaged, summarised, and made relevant to clinicians further action will be needed to ensure their implementation.

A complex set of factors influences the uptake of research findings, and a variety of dissemination methods need to be used to encourage clinicians to make informed changes in their practice.[29] Much research on effective implementation is currently under way, but a nationally coordinated strategy to disseminate and promote important evidence from research and systematic reviews could improve implementation among healthcare professionals. National campaigns to distribute information packs, briefings, and videos of important points from research findings could speed the wider adoption of changes in practice. Such national campaigns would need to be complemented by a variety of other activities at a local level.[30] Local implementation strategies involving continuing education programmes, patient education programmes, and library and information outreach services could be coordinated to ensure that key research evidence is not only accessible but also acted on.

The articles in this series are adapted from *Getting research findings into practice*, edited by Andrew Haines and Anna Donald, which is published by the BMJ Publishing Group.

▶ Acknowledgments

Helpful comments were provided by Olwen Jones, Susan Mottram, Ian Watt, Trevor Sheldon, Andrew Jones, and the two referees for this paper.

Funding: None.

Conflict of interest: None.

▶ References

1. NHS Executive. *Priorities and planning guidance for the NHS: 1997/98.* Leeds: Department of Health, 1996.
2. Glasziou PP. Support for trials of promising medications through the pharmaceutical benefits scheme: a proposal for a new authority category. *Med J Aust* 1995; **162**: 33–36 .
3. Stern K. Clinical guidelines and negligence liability. In: Deighan M, Hitch S, eds. *Clinical effectiveness from guidelines to cost-effective practice.* Brentwood: Earlybrave Publications, 1995.
4. Doctors in the dock. *Economist* 1995;**Aug 19**:23–4.
5. URL: http://biomednet.com/.
6. Dickersin K, Scherer R, Lefebvre C. Identifying relevant studies for systematic reviews. *BMJ* 1994; **309**: 1286–1291.
7. McKibbon KA, Wilczynski NL, Walker-Dilks CJ. How to search for and find evidence about therapy. *Evidence-Based Medicine* 1996; **1**: 70–72.
8. Oxman AD. Checklists for review articles. *BMJ* 1994; **309**: 648–651.
9. Hayward RS, Wilson MC, Tunis SR, Bass EB, Guyatt GH. How to use clinical practice guidelines. Part A. Are the recommendations valid? *JAMA* 1995; **274**: 570–574.
10. Wilson MC, Hayward RS, Tunis SR, Bass EB, Guyatt GH. How to use clinical practice guidelines. Part B. What are the results and will they help me in caring for my patients? *JAMA* 1995; **274**: 1630–1632.
11. URL: http://www.nlm.nih.gov/databases/freemedl.html.
12. Kuller AB, Wessel CB, Ginn DS, Martin TP. Quality filtering of the clinical literature by librarians and physicians. *Bull Med Libr Assoc* 1993; **81**: 38–43.
13. Marshall JG. The impact of the hospital library on clinical decision-making: the Rochester study. *Bull Med Libr Assoc* 1992; **80**: 169–178.
14. Klein MS, Ross FV, Adams DL, Gilbert CM. Effects of on-line literature searching on length of stay and patient care costs. *Acad Med* 1994; **69**: 489–495.
15. Urquhart CJ, Hepworth JB. The value to clinical decision making of information supplied by NHS Library and Information Services. London: British Library, 1995 (British Library research and development report no. 6205.)
16. Cimpl K. Clinical medical librarianship: a review of the literature. *Bull Med Libr Assoc* 1985; **73**: 21–28.
17. Schatz CA, Whitehead SE. "Librarian for hire": contracting a librarian's services to external departments. *Bull Med Libr Assoc* 1995; **83**: 469–472.
18. Wallingford KT, Ruffin AB, Ginter KA, Spann ML, Johnson FE, Dutcher GA, et al. Outreach activities of the National Library of Medicine: a five-year review. *Bull Med Libr Assoc*
19. Rowlands JK, Forrester WH, McSean T. British Medical Association library free Medline service: survey of members taking part in an initial pilot project. *Bull Med Libr Assoc* 1996;**84**:116–21.
20. URL: http://wwwlib.jr2.ox.ac.uk/prise/.
21. Palmer J, Streatfield D. Good diagnosis for the twenty-first century. *Libr Assoc Rec* 1995; **97**: 153–154.
22. URL: http://www.nlm.nih.gov/nichsr/nichsr.html .

23. Scottish intercollegiate guidelines network. *Clinical guidelines: criteria for appraisal for national use.* Edinburgh: SIGN, 1995.
24. NHS Executive. *Improving outcomes in breast cancer: the research evidence.* London: Department of Health, 1996.
25. http://hiru.mcmaster.ca/cpg/.
26. Oliver S, Rajan L, Turner H, Oakley A. *A pilot study of "Informed Choice" leaflets on positions in labour and routine ultrasound.* York: NHS Centre for Reviews and Dissemination, 1996.
27. Spiers PS, Guntheroth WG. Recommendations to avoid the prone sleeping position and recent statistics for sudden infant death syndrome in the United States. *Arch Pediatr Adolesc Med* 1994; **148**: 141–146.
28. Hilley CM, Morley CJ. Evaluation of government's campaign to reduce risk of cot death. *BMJ* 1994; **309**: 703–704.
29. Deykin D, Haines A. Promoting the use of research findings. In: Peckham M, Smith R, eds. *Scientific basis for health services.* London: BMJ Publishing Group, 1996.
30. Davis DA, Thomson MA, Oxman AD, Haynes RB. Changing physician performance: a systematic review of the effect of continuing medical education strategies. *JAMA* 1995; **274**: 700–705.

Papers that report drug trials (randomised controlled trials of therapy)

BACKGROUND

It is now well established that the evaluation of interventions (such as drug therapies, surgical operations or complex educational or behavioural treatments) should be undertaken as far as possible by means of double-blind, randomised controlled trials (RCTs).

SUGGESTED AIM FOR THIS SESSION

For participants to develop, and feel confident in helping others to develop, the ability to determine whether the results and conclusions of a research article advocating (or dismissing) a specific intervention are valid and applicable to their own practice and to address issues of implementation of research evidence using their findings.

SUGGESTED LEARNING OBJECTIVES FOR THIS SESSION

By the end of this session, participants should be able to:
* confirm that a paper described as a RCT actually involved adequately concealed random allocation of trial participants;
* establish whether the trial addressed an important and relevant question;
* assess the methodological quality of the RCT using a structured checklist;
* assess the significance of the results in terms of quantified measures of benefit and harm;
* comment critically on the application and implementation of the results.

SET ARTICLE

UK Prospective Diabetes Study Group. Tight blood pressure control and risk of macrovascular and microvascular complications in type 2 diabetes: UKPDS 38. *BMJ* 1999; **317**: 703–13.

ADDITIONAL REPRINT

Kunz R, Oxman AD. The unpredictability paradox: review of empirical comparisons of randomised and non-randomised clinical trials. *BMJ* 1998; **317**: 1185–90.

Clinical scenario

You are a multidisciplinary team working to develop a Health Improvement Plan for diabetes in a population of about 100 000. The group comprises a consultant diabetologist, a general physician, a consultant in public health, an optometrist, a podiatrist, a diabetes specialist nurse, a practice nurse, a pharmacist, a clinical effectiveness coordinator, and two patient representatives. One of the patient representatives has had great problems with recurrent "hypos" after her GP changed her oral medication; the other has no symptoms whatsoever but has heard that even in the absence of symptoms, the diabetes can do damage.

SUGGESTIONS FOR GROUP EXERCISES

When you have read the paper, try one or more of the following:
1. A role play in which members of your group represent these different health professionals at a meeting to decide the aims of treatment for people with diabetes.
2. A teaching situation in which some final-year medical or nursing students are asked to appraise the paper.
3. An interview with a lay newspaper for diabetes patients and their carers in which a journalist with no detailed medical knowledge is asking you to explain the findings of the study.

SUGGESTION FOR INDIVIDUAL STUDY

Imagine you are a person with type 2 diabetes. Your HbA1c level was 7.5% at the last check-up (normal laboratory range 3.5–5.5%). Your blood pressure is consistently around 164/94. Your doctor tells you that you must control your blood sugar levels more tightly, take tablets for your blood pressure, stop smoking, go to the gym, and follow a strict diet. You decide to try to find out how much benefit you can expect to gain from any or all of these changes.

You ask a friend who is a medical librarian to look out for some papers and she produces four or five key references, one of which is the UKPDS study reprinted here. If you felt you had to choose between taking treatment for your blood pressure and improving your blood glucose control, which would you choose, and why? How would you persuade your doctor of your arguments?

FURTHER READING

Greenhalgh T. *How to read a paper: the basics of evidence-based medicine*. London: BMJ Books, 1997. See in particular Chapter 3: Getting your bearings, pages 34–52 and Chapter 6: Papers that report drug trials, pages 87–96.

Guyatt GH, Sackett DL, Cook DJ. Users' guides to the medical literature. II. How to use an article about therapy or prevention. A. Are the results of the study valid? *JAMA* 1993; **270**: 2598–601.

Guyatt GH, Sackett DL, Cook DJ. Users' guides to the medical literature. II. How to use an article about therapy or prevention. B. What were the results and will they help me in caring for my patients? *JAMA* 1994; **271**: 59–63.

**CRITICAL APPRAISAL CHECKLIST FOR AN ARTICLE
DESCRIBING A RANDOMISED CONTROLLED TRIAL**

Note that the questions on the checklist are really looking for problems of bias, confounding, low power, and poor validity.

A. Are the results of the trial valid?	Yes/No/Don't know
1. Did the trial address a clearly focused question (PIO)? • Population • Intervention • Outcome	
2. Were patients randomly selected from a defined population?	
3. Was the assignment of patients to the intervention and control group randomised?	
4. Were participants and observers both "blinded" to which group they were in, control or experimental? • If not, were they single blinded (either observer or participant is blinded to allocation)? Would double blinding have been technically possible? • If not blinded at all, would blinding (single or double) have been possible?	
5. Aside from the intervention, were the two groups treated equally?	
6. Did the study have adequate power to see an effect if there was one?	
7. Were all the patients who entered the trial properly accounted for? • Was follow-up > 80%? • Were patients analysed in the groups to which they were randomised?	
B. What are the results?	
8. How large was the effect of treatment? • What outcomes were measured (measures of risk)?	
9. How precise was the estimate of the treatment effect? • Confidence intervals, p-values	
C. How relevant are the results?	
10. Were the study participants sufficiently different from my patient that this study doesn't help me at all?	

Tight blood pressure control and risk of macrovascular and microvascular complications in type 2 diabetes: UKPDS 38

UK Prospective Diabetes Study Group

Abstract

Objective: To determine whether tight control of blood pressure prevents macrovascular and microvascular complications in patients with type 2 diabetes.

Design: Randomised controlled trial comparing tight control of blood pressure aiming at a blood pressure of < 150/85 mm Hg (with the use of an angiotensin converting enzyme inhibitor captopril or a β blocker atenolol as main treatment) with less tight control aiming at a blood pressure of < 180/105 mm Hg.

Setting: 20 hospital based clinics in England, Scotland, and Northern Ireland.

Subjects: 1148 hypertensive patients with type 2 diabetes (mean age 56, mean blood pressure at entry 160/94 mm Hg); 758 patients were allocated to tight control of blood pressure and 390 patients to less tight control with a median follow up of 8.4 years.

Main outcome measures: Predefined clinical end points, fatal and non-fatal, related to diabetes, deaths related to diabetes, and all cause mortality. Surrogate measures of microvascular disease included urinary albumin excretion and retinal photography.

Results: Mean blood pressure during follow up was significantly reduced in the group assigned tight blood pressure control (144/82 mm Hg) compared with the group assigned to less tight control (154/87 mm Hg) (P < 0.0001). Reductions in risk in the group assigned to tight control compared with that assigned to less tight control were 24% in diabetes related end points (95% confidence interval 8% to 38%) (P = 0.0046), 32% in deaths related to diabetes (6% to 51%) (P = 0.019), 44% in strokes (11% to 65%) (P = 0.013), and 37% in microvascular end points (11% to 56%) (P = 0.0092), predominantly owing to a reduced risk of retinal photocoagulation. There was a non-significant reduction in all cause mortality. After nine years of follow up the group assigned to tight blood pressure control also had a 34% reduction in risk in the proportion of patients with deterioration of retinopathy by two steps (99% confidence interval 11% to 50%) (P = 0.0004) and a 47% reduced risk (7% to 70%) (P = 0.004) of deterioration in visual acuity by three lines of the early treatment of diabetic retinopathy study (ETDRS) chart. After nine years of follow up 29% of patients in the group assigned to tight control required three or more treatments to lower blood pressure to achieve target blood pressures.

Conclusion: Tight blood pressure control in patients with hypertension and type 2 diabetes achieves a clinically important reduction in the risk of deaths related to diabetes, complications related to diabetes, progression of diabetic retinopathy, and deterioration in visual acuity.

Introduction

Type 2 diabetes and hypertension are commonly associated conditions, both of which carry an increased risk of cardiovascular and renal disease.[1-6] The prevalence of hypertension in type 2 diabetes is higher than that in the general population, especially in younger patients.[7-9] At the age of 45 around 40% of patients with type 2 diabetes are hypertensive, the proportion increasing to 60% by the age of 75.[7-9] Hypertension increases the already high risk of cardiovascular disease associated with type 2 diabetes[2 3 6 10] and is also a risk factor for the development of microalbuminuria[11 12] and retinopathy.[13]

In the general population treatment to lower blood pressure reduces the incidence of stroke and myocardial infarction,[14 15] particularly in elderly people.[16 17] In patients with type 1 diabetes who have microalbuminuria or overt nephropathy strict control of blood pressure reduces urinary albumin excretion and deterioration in renal function.[18 19] Lowering blood pressure also decreases albuminuria in type 2 diabetes,[20] but whether it also reduces the risk of end stage renal disease or of cardiac disease is not known.

We report results from the hypertension in diabetes study, a multicentre, randomised, controlled trial (embedded within the UK prospective diabetes study) designed to determine whether tight blood pressure control (aiming for a blood pressure of < 150/85 mm Hg) reduces morbidity and mortality in hypertensive patients with type 2 diabetes.[21]

Subjects and methods

We studied hypertensive patients with type 2 diabetes who had been recruited to the UK prospective diabetes study.[22 23] General practitioners were asked to refer

Originally published in *BMJ* 1998; **317**: 703–13.

Editorials by Orchard and Mogensen
Papers pp 713, 720

Members of the study group are given at the end of the paper.

This paper was prepared for publication by Robert Turner, Rury Holman, Irene Stratton, Carole Cull, Valeria Frighi, Susan Manley, David Matthews, Andrew Neil, Heather McElroy, Eva Kohner, Charles Fox, David Hadden, and David Wright.

Correspondence to: Professor R Turner, UK Prospective Diabetes Study Group, Diabetes Research Laboratories, Radcliffe Infirmary, Oxford OX2 6HE

BMJ 1998;317:703–13

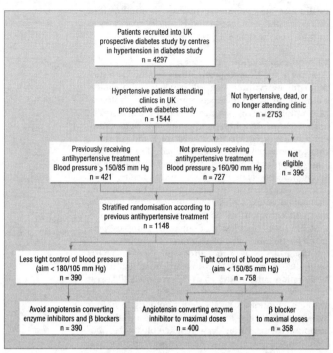

Fig 1 Selection and random allocation of patients to treatment in hypertension in diabetes study

patients aged 25-65 with newly diagnosed diabetes to 23 participating centres. A total of 5102 were recruited as they met the study's entry criterion (fasting plasma glucose concentration >6 mmol/l on two mornings), were willing to join, and did not meet the exclusion criteria for the study. Exclusion criteria were ketonuria >3 mmol/l; a history of myocardial infarction in the previous year; current angina or heart failure; more than one major vascular episode; serum creatinine concentration >175 µmol/l; retinopathy requiring laser treatment; malignant hypertension; an uncorrected endocrine abnormality; an occupation which would preclude insulin treatment (such as heavy goods vehicle driver); a severe concurrent illness likely to limit life or require extensive systemic treatment; or inadequate understanding or unwillingness to enter the study.[22 23] The patients were treated by diet alone for 3 months.[24] Patients who remained hyperglycaemic (fasting plasma glucose 6.1-15.0 mmol/l) without diabetic symptoms were randomly allocated conventional blood glucose control, primarily by diet, or intensive control (aiming for a fasting plasma glucose concentration <6.0 mmol/l) with additional sulphonylurea, insulin, or metformin treatment. Details of the protocol are published.[22 23]

Of the 4297 patients recruited to the 20 centres participating in the hypertension in diabetes study, 243 had either died or were lost to follow up before the start of the hypertension study in 1987 (fig 1). Of the remaining 4054 patients, 1544 (38%) had hypertension, defined in 727 patients as a systolic blood pressure ≥160 mm Hg and/or a diastolic blood pressure ≥90 mm Hg or in 421 patients receiving antihypertensive treatment as a systolic pressure of ≥150 mm Hg and/or a diastolic pressure ≥85 mm Hg (fig 1). Patients were enrolled on the basis of the mean

of three blood pressure measurements taken at consecutive clinic visits. The exclusion criteria were a clinical requirement for strict blood pressure control (previous stroke, accelerated hypertension, cardiac failure, or renal failure) or β blockade (myocardial infarction in the previous year or current angina); severe vascular disease (more than one major vascular episode); a severe concurrent illness or contraindications to β blockers (asthma, intermittent claudication, foot ulcers, or amputations); pregnancy; or unwillingness to join the study. Of the 1544 hypertensive patients, 252 were excluded and 144 patients did not enter the study. A total of 1148 patients (637 men (55%)) with a mean age of 56.4 (SD 8.1) years entered the hypertension in diabetes study between 1987 and 1991.[21] Table 1 shows their characteristics at randomisation to blood pressure control policy.

Table 1 Characteristics of patients allocated to tight and less tight control of blood pressure. Values are numbers (percentages) of patients unless stated otherwise

	Tight (n=758)	Less tight (n=390)
Mean (SD) age (years)	56.4 (8.1)	56.5 (8.1)
Male sex	410 (54)	227 (58)
Ethnic group:		
White	651 (86)	344 (88)
Afro Caribbean	62 (8)	25 (6)
Asian Indian	39 (5)	17 (4)
Other	6 (1)	4 (1)
Mean (SD) body mass index (kg/m²)	29.8 (5.5)	29.3 (5.5)
Median (interquartile range) fasting plasma glucose (mmol/l)	7.4 (6.1 to 9.2)	7.4 (6.2 to 9.8)
Mean (SD) haemoglobin A₁c (%)	6.9 (1.7)	6.8 (1.5)
Mean (SD) blood pressure (mm Hg):		
Systolic	159 (20)	160 (18)
Diastolic	94 (10)	94 (9)
Receiving antihypertensive treatment	286 (36)	145 (37)
Smoking:		
No of patients	746	379
Non smoker	281 (38)	142 (38)
Ex smoker	294 (39)	152 (40)
Current smoker	171 (23)	85 (22)
Urinary albumin (mg/l)*:		
≥50	114 (18)	53 (16)
≥300	18 (3)	13 (4)
Retinopathy:		
No of patients	617	312
20 20 or worse	143 (23)	89 (29)
35 35 or worse	45 (7)	32 (10)
Mean (SD) cholesterol (mmol/l):		
Total	5.5 (1.1)	5.6 (1.1)
HDL	1.10 (0.27)	1.10 (0.28)
LDL	3.6 (1.1)	3.6 (1.1)
Geometric mean (1SD interval) triglyceride (mmol/l)	1.6 (0.9 to 2.6)	1.6 (0.9 to 2.8)
Median duration (interquartile range) of diabetes (years)	2.7 (1.0 to 4.2)	2.5 (1.0 to 4.4)
Treatment for diabetes:		
Diet	175 (29)	89 (29)
Sulphonylurea	200 (34)	103 (34)
Metformin	41 (8)	23 (7)
Combined oral hypoglycaemic agents	28 (5)	16 (5)
Insulin	144 (23)	70 (24)
Other	6 (1)	1 (1)

HDL=high density lipoprotein.
LDL=low density lipoprotein.
*Corrected to urinary creatinine concentration of 8 mmol/l.

Treatment protocol

Randomisation stratified for those with or without previous treatment for hypertension was performed by the coordinating centre. In all 758 patients were allocated tight control of blood pressure, aiming for a blood pressure <150/85 mm Hg (400 patients were given an angiotensin converting enzyme inhibitor (captopril) and 358 a β blocker (atenolol) as the main treatment); 390 patients were allocated a less tight control of blood pressure, aiming for a blood pressure <180/105 mm Hg but avoiding treatment with angiotensin converting enzyme inhibitors or β blockers (fig 1). Sealed opaque envelopes were used and checked as described for the UK prospective diabetes study.[23] The original blood pressure target of 200/105 mm Hg in the group assigned to less tight control was reduced in 1992 by the steering committee of the hypertension in diabetes study after publication of the results of studies in elderly, non-diabetic subjects during 1991-2.[16 25 26] Randomisation produced balanced numbers of patients allocated to the various glucose and blood pressure treatment combinations for the UK prospective diabetes study and hypertension in diabetes study.

Captopril was usually started at a dose of 25 mg twice daily, increasing to 50 mg twice daily, and atenolol at a daily dose of 50 mg, increasing to 100 mg if required. Other agents were added if the control criteria were not met in the group assigned to tight control despite maximum allocated treatment or in the group assigned to less tight control without drug treatment. The suggested sequence was frusemide 20 mg daily (maximum 40 mg twice daily), slow release nifedipine 10 mg (maximum 40 mg) twice daily, methyldopa 250 mg (maximum 500 mg) twice daily, and prazosin 1 mg (maximum 5 mg) thrice daily.

Clinic visits

Patients visited study clinics every 3-4 months. At each visit plasma glucose concentration, blood pressure, and body weight were measured, and treatments to control blood pressure and blood glucose concentration were noted and adjusted if target values were not met. If treatments and target blood pressures were not in accord with the protocol, the coordinating centre sent letters about affected patients to the clinical centres requesting appropriate action. A central record of all apparent protocol deviations was maintained. Symptoms including any drug side effects and clinical events were noted. Physicians recorded hypoglycaemic episodes as minor if the patient was able to treat the symptoms unaided and as major if third party or medical intervention was necessary.

Blood pressure measurements

Blood pressure (diastolic phase 5) while the patient was sitting and had rested for at least five minutes was measured by a trained nurse with a Copal UA-251 or a Takeda UA-751 electronic auscultatory blood pressure reading machine (Andrew Stephens, Brighouse, West Yorkshire) or with a Hawksley random zero sphygmomanometer (Hawksley, Lancing, Sussex) in patients with atrial fibrillation. The first reading was discarded and the mean of the next three consecutive readings with a coefficient of variation below 15% was used in the study, with additional readings if required. Monthly quality assurance measurements have shown the mean difference between Takeda and Hawksley machines to be 1 (4) mm Hg or less.

Clinical examination

At entry to the UK prospective diabetes study and subsequently every three years all patients had a clinical examination which included retinal colour photography, ophthalmoscopy, measurement of visual acuity, assessment of peripheral and autonomic neuropathy, chest radiography, electrocardiography, and measurement of brachial and posterior tibial blood pressure using Doppler techniques. Annual direct ophthalmoscopy was also carried out. Every year a fasting blood sample was taken to measure glycated haemoglobin (haemoglobin A_{1c}), plasma creatinine concentration, and concentrations of urea, immunoreactive insulin, and insulin antibodies; random urine samples were taken for measurement of albumin concentration.

Visual acuity was measured with Snellen charts until 1989, after which ETDRS (early treatment of diabetic retinopathy study) charts[22] were used to assess best corrected vision, with current refraction or through a pinhole. Retinal colour photographs of four standard 30° fields per eye (nasal, disc, macula, and temporal to macular fields) were taken plus stereophotographs of the macula. Repeat photography was arranged if the quality of the photograph was unsatisfactory. Retinal photographs were assessed at a central grading centre by two independent assessors for the presence or absence of diabetic retinopathy. Any fields with retinopathy were graded by two further senior independent assessors using a modified ETDRS final scale.[22] Neuropathy was assessed clinically by knee and ankle reflexes, and by biothesiometer (Biomedical Instruments, Newbury, Ohio) readings taken from the lateral malleoli and the end of the big toe.[22] A 12 lead electrocardiogram was recorded and given a Minnesota code,[22] and a chest x ray film was taken for measurement of cardiac diameter.

Biochemistry

Biochemical methods have been reported previously.[23 27] Urinary albumin concentration was measured by an immunoturbidimetric method with a normal reference range of 1.4 mg/l to 36.5 mg/l.[27] Microalbuminuria has been defined as a urinary albumin concentration of ≥50 mg/l[28] and clinical grade proteinuria as a urinary albumin concentration of ≥300 mg/l.

Clinical end points

Twenty one clinical end points were predefined in the study protocol.[22] All available clinical information was gathered for possible end points—for example, copies of admission notes, operation records, death certificates, and necropsy reports. Copies of these, without reference to the patient's allocated or actual treatment, were formally presented to two independent physicians who allocated an appropriate code from the ninth revision of the international classification of diseases (ICD-9) if the criteria for any particular clinical end point had been met. Any disagreement between the two assessors was discussed and the evidence reviewed. If agreement was not possible the information was submitted to a panel of two further independent assessors for final arbitration. The closing date for the study was 30 September 1997.

End points were aggregated for the main analyses. The three predefined primary outcome analyses were the time to the occurrence of (*a*) a first clinical end point related to diabetes (sudden death, death from hyperglycaemia or hypoglycaemia, fatal or non-fatal myocardial infarction, angina, heart failure, stroke, renal failure, amputation (of at least one digit), vitreous haemorrhage, retinal photocoagulation, blindness in one eye or cataract extraction); (*b*) death related to diabetes (death due to myocardial infarction, sudden death, stroke, peripheral vascular disease, renal disease, hyperglycaemia or hypoglycaemia); (*c*) death from all causes.

Secondary outcome analyses of four additional aggregates of clinical end points were used to assess the effect of treatments on different types of vascular disease. These were myocardial infarction (fatal or non-fatal myocardial infarction or sudden death), stroke (fatal or non-fatal stroke), amputation or death from peripheral vascular disease, and microvascular complications (retinopathy requiring photocoagulation, vitreous haemorrhage, and fatal or non-fatal renal failure).

Since a patient could in sequence have different end points, he or she could be included in more than one end point category.

Surrogate end points—Details of subclinical, surrogate variables have been published.[23]

Statistical analysis

Analysis was on an intention to treat basis, comparing patients allocated to tight and less tight blood pressure control. Patients allocated to tight control with angiotensin converting enzyme inhibitors or β blockers were pooled in this paper for analysis. They are compared in the accompanying paper.[29] Life table analyses were performed with log rank tests, and hazard ratios were obtained from Cox's proportional hazards models and used to estimate relative risks. Survival function estimates were calculated using the product limit (Kaplan-Meier) method. In the text relative risks are quoted as risk reductions and significance tests were two sided. For aggregate end points 95% confidence intervals are quoted, whereas for single end points 99% confidence intervals are quoted to allow for potential type 1 errors. Similarly, 99% confidence intervals were used to assess surrogate end points that were measured at triennial visits. Mean (SD), geometric mean (1 SD interval), or median (interquartile range) values are quoted for the biometric and biochemical variables, with values from Wilcoxon, *t*, or χ^2 tests for comparisons. Risk reductions for surrogate end points were derived from frequency tables. The overall values for blood pressure during a period were assessed for each patient as the mean during that period and for each allocation as the mean of patients with data in the allocation. Control of blood pressure was assessed in patients allocated to the two groups who had data at nine years of follow up.

Hypoglycaemia was determined from the number of patients allocated to a treatment and continuing with it who had one or more minor or major hypoglycaemic episodes each year. Urinary albumin concentration was measured in mg/l. Change in

diabetic retinopathy was defined as a change of two steps (one step in both eyes or two or more steps in one eye) with a scale from the worse eye to the better eye that included retinal photocoagulation or vitreous haemorrhage as the most serious grade. Visual loss was defined as the best vision in either eye, deteriorating by three lines on an ETDRS chart.

Both the UK prospective diabetes study and hypertension in diabetes study received ethical approval from the appropriate committee in each centre and conformed with the guidelines of the Declarations of Helsinki (1975 and 1983). All patients gave informed consent.

Data monitoring and ethics committee

The data monitoring and ethics committee examined the end points every six months to consider halting or modifying the study according to predetermined guidelines. These included a difference of three or more standard deviations by log rank test in the rate of deaths related to diabetes or deaths related to diabetes and major illness between the group assigned to tight control and that assigned to less tight control or between the group given captopril and that given atenolol.[22] One of the stopping criteria was attained immediately before the scheduled end of the study.

Results

Follow up

The median follow up to death, the last known date at which vital status was known, or to the end of the trial was 8.4 years. The vital status was known at the end of the trial in all patients except 14 (1%) who had emigrated and a further 33 patients (3%) who could not be contacted in the last year of the study for assessment of clinical end points.

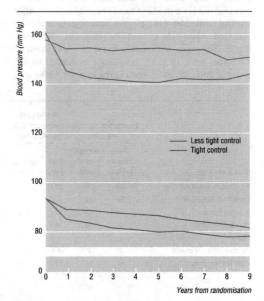

Fig 2 Mean systolic and diastolic blood pressures over nine years in 297 patients in group assigned to tight control of blood pressure and 156 in group assigned to less tight control

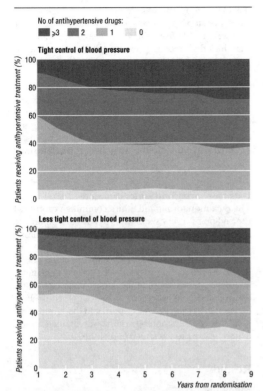

No of antihypertensive drugs:
▮ >3 ▮ 2 ▮ 1 ▯ 0

Fig 3 Proportion of patients over nine years who required no drugs, one drug, two drugs, or three or more drugs for treating hypertension to attain target blood pressure

Control of blood pressure

The mean (SD) blood pressure in the two groups was similar at randomisation (table 1). Mean blood pressure in patients over nine years of follow up was 144 (14)/82 (7) mm Hg in the 297 patients under tight control and 154 (16)/87 (7) mm Hg in the 156 assigned to less tight control (P<0.0001 in both cases) (fig 2). The mean differences in systolic and diastolic pressures were 10 (95% confidence interval 9 to 12) mm Hg and 5 (4 to 6) mm Hg respectively. Cross sec-

tional blood pressure in patients with data at each year were similar to the data in patients with nine years of follow up. At nine years the proportion of patients with both a systolic blood pressure of <150 mm Hg and a diastolic blood pressure of <85 mm Hg was 56% in the group assigned to tight control and 37% in the group assigned to less tight control. The proportion of patients who had a mean blood pressure of <180/105 mm Hg was 96% and 91% respectively.

Compliance with allocated treatment
In the group assigned to tight control of blood pressure patients took their allocated treatment for 77% of the total person years and did not take antihypertensive treatments for 6% of the total person years. In the other group patients did not take any antihypertensive treatments for 43% of the total person years; they took an angiotensin converting enzyme inhibitor for 11% of the total person years and a β blocker for 9%.

Figure 3 shows the increasing number of antihypertensive agents required to maintain blood pressure lower than target levels. At nine years 29% of those assigned to tight blood pressure control required three or more agents in comparison with 11% of patients in the other group. The proportion of patients taking nifedipine was 32% in the group assigned to less tight blood pressure control and 31% and 40% in the group assigned to tight blood pressure control taking captopril and atenolol respectively.

Control of blood glucose
Haemoglobin A_{1c} in the groups assigned to tight and less tight blood pressure control over 1-4 years was 7.2% and 7.2% respectively and over 5-8 years 8.3% and 8.2% respectively.

Aggregate clinical end points

Any clinical end point related to diabetes
Patients allocated to tight compared with less tight control of blood pressure had a 24% reduction in risk of developing any end point related to diabetes, (P=0.0046) (figs 4 and 5).

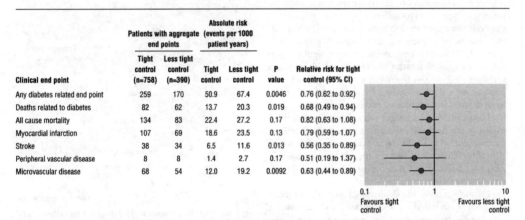

Clinical end point	Patients with aggregate end points		Absolute risk (events per 1000 patient years)		P value	Relative risk for tight control (95% CI)
	Tight control (n=758)	Less tight control (n=390)	Tight control	Less tight control		
Any diabetes related end point	259	170	50.9	67.4	0.0046	0.76 (0.62 to 0.92)
Deaths related to diabetes	82	62	13.7	20.3	0.019	0.68 (0.49 to 0.94)
All cause mortality	134	83	22.4	27.2	0.17	0.82 (0.63 to 1.08)
Myocardial infarction	107	69	18.6	23.5	0.13	0.79 (0.59 to 1.07)
Stroke	38	34	6.5	11.6	0.013	0.56 (0.35 to 0.89)
Peripheral vascular disease	8	8	1.4	2.7	0.17	0.51 (0.19 to 1.37)
Microvascular disease	68	54	12.0	19.2	0.0092	0.63 (0.44 to 0.89)

Fig 4 Numbers of patients who attained one or more clinical end points in aggregates representing specific types of clinical complications, with relative risks comparing tight control of blood pressure with less tight control

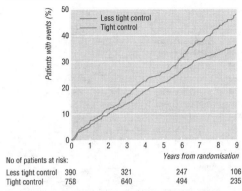

No of patients at risk:

Less tight control	390	321	247	106
Tight control	758	640	494	235

Reduction in risk with tight control 24% (95% CI 8% to 38%)(P = 0.0046)

Fig 5 Kaplan Meier plots of proportions of patients with any clinical end point, fatal or non fatal, related to diabetes

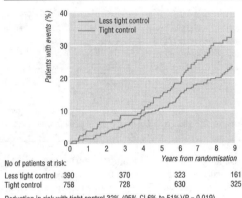

No of patients at risk:

Less tight control	390	370	323	161
Tight control	758	728	630	325

Reduction in risk with tight control 32% (95% CI 6% to 51%)(P = 0.019)

Fig 6 Kaplan Meier plots of proportions of patients who die of disease related to diabetes (myocardial infarction, sudden death, stroke, peripheral vascular disease, and renal failure)

Deaths related to diabetes and all cause mortality
Patients in the group assigned to tight blood pressure control compared with those in the other group had a 32% reduction in risk of mortality from diseases substantially increased by diabetes (P=0.019), two thirds of which were cardiovascular diseases. The reduction in all cause mortality was not significant (fig 4). The trend to protection against microvascular disease and death related to diabetes became evident within the first three years of allocation to tight control (figs 4-7).

Myocardial infarction, stroke and peripheral vascular disease
The group assigned to tight blood pressure control had a non-significant reduction in risk of 21% in the aggregate end point for myocardial infarction (table 2 and fig 7). This group also had a 44% reduction in risk of stroke, fatal and non-fatal, compared with the group assigned to less tight blood pressure control (P=0.013). Amputations were not significantly reduced, with a trend to reductions in risk of 49%. One patient in each group died of peripheral vascular disease.

When all macrovascular diseases were combined, including myocardial infarction, sudden death, stroke,

and peripheral vascular disease, the group assigned to tight blood pressure control had a 34% reduction in risk compared with the group assigned to less tight control (P = 0.019).

Microvascular disease
The group assigned to tight blood pressure control had a 37% reduction in risk of microvascular disease compared with the less tight group (P = 0.0092) (figs 4 and 7).

Numbers needed to treat
The number of patients who needed to be treated over 10 years to prevent one patient developing any complication was 6.1 (95% confidence interval 2.6 to 9.5) and to prevent death from a cause related to diabetes 15.0 (12.1 to 17.9).

Single clinical end points
There was a 56% reduction in risk of heart failure (P = 0.0043) (fig 8) in the tight control group compared with the less tight control group. There was a 35% reduction in risk of retinal photocoagulation

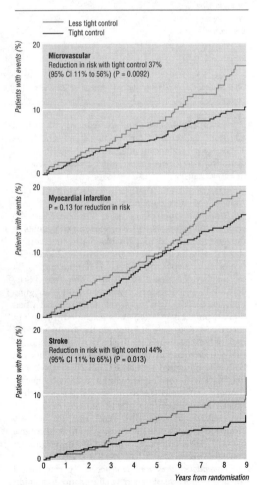

Fig 7 Kaplan Meier plots of proportions of patients who developed microvascular end points (mostly retinal photocoagulation), fatal or non fatal myocardial infarction or sudden death, and fatal or non fatal strokes

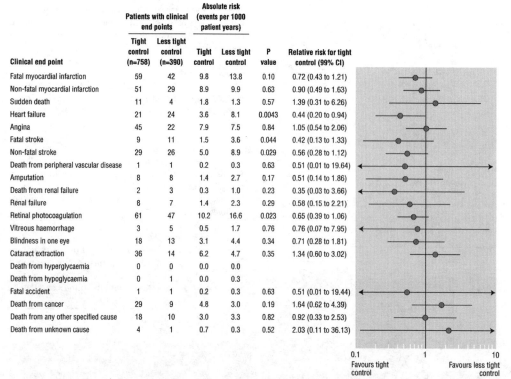

Clinical end point	Patients with clinical end points		Absolute risk (events per 1000 patient years)		P value	Relative risk for tight control (99% CI)
	Tight control (n=758)	Less tight control (n=390)	Tight control	Less tight control		
Fatal myocardial infarction	59	42	9.8	13.8	0.10	0.72 (0.43 to 1.21)
Non-fatal myocardial infarction	51	29	8.9	9.9	0.63	0.90 (0.49 to 1.63)
Sudden death	11	4	1.8	1.3	0.57	1.39 (0.31 to 6.26)
Heart failure	21	24	3.6	8.1	0.0043	0.44 (0.20 to 0.94)
Angina	45	22	7.9	7.5	0.84	1.05 (0.54 to 2.06)
Fatal stroke	9	11	1.5	3.6	0.044	0.42 (0.13 to 1.33)
Non-fatal stroke	29	26	5.0	8.9	0.029	0.56 (0.28 to 1.12)
Death from peripheral vascular disease	1	1	0.2	0.3	0.63	0.51 (0.01 to 19.64)
Amputation	8	8	1.4	2.7	0.17	0.51 (0.14 to 1.86)
Death from renal failure	2	3	0.3	1.0	0.23	0.35 (0.03 to 3.66)
Renal failure	8	7	1.4	2.3	0.29	0.58 (0.15 to 2.21)
Retinal photocoagulation	61	47	10.2	16.6	0.023	0.65 (0.39 to 1.06)
Vitreous haemorrhage	3	5	0.5	1.7	0.76	0.76 (0.07 to 7.95)
Blindness in one eye	18	13	3.1	4.4	0.34	0.71 (0.28 to 1.81)
Cataract extraction	36	14	6.2	4.7	0.35	1.34 (0.60 to 3.02)
Death from hyperglycaemia	0	0	0.0	0.0		
Death from hypoglycaemia	0	1	0.0	0.3		
Fatal accident	1	1	0.2	0.3	0.63	0.51 (0.01 to 19.44)
Death from cancer	29	9	4.8	3.0	0.19	1.64 (0.62 to 4.39)
Death from any other specified cause	18	10	3.0	3.3	0.82	0.92 (0.33 to 2.53)
Death from unknown cause	4	1	0.7	0.3	0.52	2.03 (0.11 to 36.13)

Fig 8 Numbers of patients who attained individual end points, with relative risks comparing tight control of blood pressure with less tight control

(P=0.023) (fig 8). The trend for reduced risk of fatal and non-fatal renal failure was non-significant (fig 8). There was no significant difference in the incidence of death from accidents, cancer, other specified causes or unknown causes.

Analyses of surrogate end points

Retinopathy and visual acuity—From median 4.5 years of follow up a smaller proportion of patients in the group assigned to tight blood pressure control showed deterioration in retinopathy from baseline by two or more steps (fig 9), with a 34% reduction in risk by median 7.5 years (P=0.004). This was partly because fewer patients required retinal photocoagulation, but the risk was still significantly reduced when retinal photocoagulation was excluded (data not shown). At nine years of follow up the group assigned to tight blood pressure control had a 47% reduction in risk of a decrease in vision by three or more lines in both eyes measured with an ETDRS chart (P=0.004) (fig 9). There was no significant difference in the proportion of patients with impaired vision preventing driving (visual acuity < 6/12 Snellen or ETDRS chart>0.3), although the trend was for a 28% reduction in risk in the group assigned to tight control (32/371, 8.6%) compared with the group assigned to less tight control (24/201,11.9%) (P=0.20).

Microalbuminuria and proteinuria—By six years a smaller proportion of patients in the group under tight blood pressure control had a urinary albumin concentration of ≥50 mg/l, a 29% reduction in risk (P=0.009), with a non-significant 39% reduction in

risk for proteinuria ≥300 mg/l (P=0.061) (fig 9). The reduction in risk for both a urinary albumin concentration of ≥50 mg/l and proteinuria at nine years of follow up was not significant. There was no significant difference in plasma creatinine concentra-

Table 2 Comparison of results of hypertension in diabetes study with those of systolic hypertension in elderly programme[29]

	Hypertension in diabetes study	Systolic hypertension in elderly programme
No of subjects	1148	583
Mean (SD) age (years)	56 (8)	70 (6)
Proportion of men (%)	55	50
Blood pressure on entry (mm Hg)	160/94	170/76
Proportion receiving antihypertensive drugs (%)	36	42
Diabetes entry criterion	Fasting plasma glucose >6 mmol/l on 2 occasions	Known diabetes or fasting plasma glucose ≥7.8 mmol/l
Hypoglycaemic treatment	Diet, oral hypoglycaemic agents, insulin	Diet, oral hypoglycaemic agents
Duration of trial (years)	9	5
Intervention in active group	Captopril or atenolol	Chlorthalidone with or without atenolol or reserpine
Blood pressure (mm Hg):		
Tight control group	144/82	145/71
Less tight control group	154/87	155/69
Difference	10/5	10/2
Outcome (relative risk (95% CI)):		
Death related to diabetes	0.68 (0.49 to 0.94)	Not reported
Myocardial infarction, fatal or non fatal, and sudden death	0.79 (0.59 to 1.07)	0.46 (0.24 to 0.88)
Stroke, fatal or non fatal	0.56 (0.35 to 0.89)	0.78 (0.45 to 1.34)
Microvascular disease	0.64 (0.44 to 0.91)	Not assessed

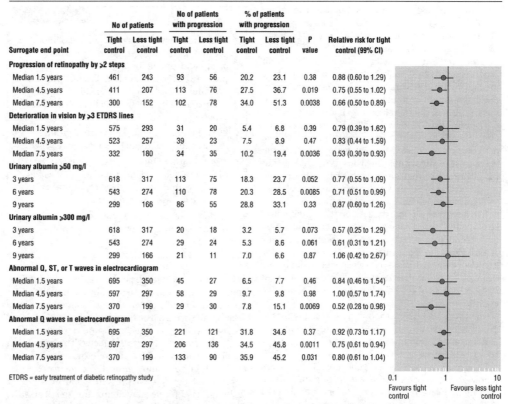

	No of patients		No of patients with progression		% of patients with progression			
Surrogate end point	Tight control	Less tight control	Tight control	Less tight control	Tight control	Less tight control	P value	Relative risk for tight control (99% CI)
Progression of retinopathy by >2 steps								
Median 1.5 years	461	243	93	56	20.2	23.1	0.38	0.88 (0.60 to 1.29)
Median 4.5 years	411	207	113	76	27.5	36.7	0.019	0.75 (0.55 to 1.02)
Median 7.5 years	300	152	102	78	34.0	51.3	0.0038	0.66 (0.50 to 0.89)
Deterioration in vision by >3 ETDRS lines								
Median 1.5 years	575	293	31	20	5.4	6.8	0.39	0.79 (0.39 to 1.62)
Median 4.5 years	523	257	39	23	7.5	8.9	0.47	0.83 (0.44 to 1.59)
Median 7.5 years	332	180	34	35	10.2	19.4	0.0036	0.53 (0.30 to 0.93)
Urinary albumin >50 mg/l								
3 years	618	317	113	75	18.3	23.7	0.052	0.77 (0.55 to 1.09)
6 years	543	274	110	78	20.3	28.5	0.0085	0.71 (0.51 to 0.99)
9 years	299	166	86	55	28.8	33.1	0.33	0.87 (0.60 to 1.26)
Urinary albumin >300 mg/l								
3 years	618	317	20	18	3.2	5.7	0.073	0.57 (0.25 to 1.29)
6 years	543	274	29	24	5.3	8.6	0.061	0.61 (0.31 to 1.21)
9 years	299	166	21	11	7.0	6.6	0.87	1.06 (0.42 to 2.67)
Abnormal Q, ST, or T waves in electrocardiogram								
Median 1.5 years	695	350	45	27	6.5	7.7	0.46	0.84 (0.46 to 1.54)
Median 4.5 years	597	297	58	29	9.7	9.8	0.98	1.00 (0.57 to 1.74)
Median 7.5 years	370	199	29	30	7.8	15.1	0.0069	0.52 (0.28 to 0.98)
Abnormal Q waves in electrocardiogram								
Median 1.5 years	695	350	221	121	31.8	34.6	0.37	0.92 (0.73 to 1.17)
Median 4.5 years	597	297	206	136	34.5	45.8	0.0011	0.75 (0.61 to 0.94)
Median 7.5 years	370	199	133	90	35.9	45.2	0.031	0.80 (0.61 to 1.04)

ETDRS = early treatment of diabetic retinopathy study

0.1   1   10
Favours tight control   Favours less tight control

Fig 9 Numbers of patients who attained surrogate end points, with relative risks comparing tight control of blood pressure with less tight control

tion or in the proportion of patients who had a twofold increase in plasma creatinine concentration between the two groups.

Neuropathy—The surrogate indices of neuropathy and autonomic neuropathy were not significantly different between the two groups.

ECG abnormality—By median 7.5 years the tight control group had a lower proportion of Q wave ECG abnormalities than the less tight control group, 29/370 and 30/199 (7.8% and 15.1%, P=0.007) respectively, a 48% risk reduction. ST and T wave abnormalities were also reduced in the tight control group (fig 9). There was no difference between the allocations for other surrogate indices of macrovascular disease.

There was no significant difference between the groups in the proportion of patients who developed surrogate indices for macrovascular disease.

Side effects

Hypoglycaemia—There was no significant difference in the cumulative incidence of hypoglycaemia in the groups assigned to tight and less tight blood pressure control, with 6.1% and 4.4% respectively having a major hypoglycaemic attack. The cause of death in one patient in the group assigned to less tight control of blood pressure was attributed to hypoglycaemia.

Weight gain—Mean weight gain was similar in the two groups (1.3 kg in the group assigned to less tight control and 2.0 kg in the tight control; P=0.13).

Discussion

This paper reports that patients with hypertension and type 2 diabetes assigned to tight control of blood pressure achieved a significant reduction in risk of 24% for any end points related to diabetes, 32% for death related to diabetes, 44% for stroke, and 37% for microvascular disease. In addition there was a 56% reduction in risk of heart failure. The mean blood pressure over nine years was 144/82mm Hg on tight control compared with a less tight control mean of 154/87mm Hg. In comparison, intensive blood glucose control in the UK prospective diabetes study decreased the risk of any diabetes related end point by 12% (P=0.029) and microvascular disease by 25% (P=0.0099).[23]

Comparison of cardiovascular results with other studies—The risk reduction for strokes is similar to results from a meta-analysis of clinical trials of improved blood pressure control in the general population, which showed risk reductions of 42% for strokes and 12% for myocardial infarction.[14] The reduction in cardiovascular end points is in accord with the results of the Systolic Hypertension in the Elderly Program for the 568 patients with non-insulin treated type 2 diabetes whose mean age was 70 and mean blood pressure 170/76mm Hg at baseline (table 2).[30] The Hypertension Optimal Treatment study showed a reduction in cardiovascular mortality for 1501 diabetic patients randomly allocated a target diastolic blood pressure of ≤80mm Hg,[31] although the blood pressures acheived have not been published. Intensive blood pressure control in the diabetic subgroup of the Hypertension Detection and Follw-up Program showed no effect on all cause mortality.[32]

Retinopathy—The was a 34% reduction in the rate of progression of retinopathy by two or more steps using the modified ETDRS final scale. The 47% reduction in the deterioration of visual acuity by three lines using the ETDRS chart (equivalent to a change from 6/6 to 6/12 or 6/9 to 6/18 on the Snellen chart) suggests that tight blood pressure control also prevented the development of diabetic maculopathy, which is the main cause of visual impairment in type 2 diabetes.[33] In the UK prospective diabetes study diabetic maculopathy occurred in 78% of patients requiring retinal photocoagulation. As diabetic maculopathy responds less well to laser retinal photocoagulation than proliferative retinopathy,[34 35] reducing the risk of maculopathy by tight blood pressure control might provide a major clinical benefit in reducing the risk of blindness. To our knowledge this is the first report in patients with type 2 diabetes to show that tight blood pressure control reduces the risk of clinical complications from diabetic eye disease.

Renal disease—The proportion of patients in the group assigned to tight blood pressure control who had a urinary albumin concentration of >50 mg/l at six years of follow up was only significantly lower than in the group assigned to less tight control at six years follow-up. Good control of blood pressure in patients with renal failure prevents progression of established renal failure in type 1 diabetes.[18 19 36] Ravid et al also showed in 49 normotensive subjects with type 2 diabetes and microalbuminuria (mean 143 mg/24 h (range 30-290)) that improved blood pressure control with enalapril prevented an increase in urine albumin excretion and gave a slower decline in renal function.[37] Previous epidemiological studies have shown an association between hypertension and albuminuria in patients with type 2 diabetes who do not have renal failure.[11 12]

High blood pressure in type 2 diabetes—Hypertension remains underrecognised and undertreated in the diabetic as well as in the general population. In the 1995 health survey for England 40% of the general population with hypertension (World Health Organisation criteria: >160 mm Hg systolic, >95 mm Hg diastolic) were not treated and one third of the treated subjects still had a blood pressure greater than 160/95 mm Hg. The mean blood pressure in the group assigned to less tight control of blood pressure in the hypertension in diabetes study over nine years of follow up from a mean age of 56 at recruitment was 154/87 mm Hg. In the second national health and nutrition survey of 1976-80 in the United States 28% of hypertensive diabetic patients had blood pressures of ≥160 mm Hg or ≥95 mm Hg.[9]

In this study the mean blood pressure in the group assigned to tight blood pressure control was 144/82 mm Hg which is lower than the blood pressures often achieved in hypertensive subjects with or without diabetes. Advisory groups have recommended that the goals for blood pressure in diabetic patients should be <140/90 mm Hg,[38-40] <140/85 mm Hg,[41] or <130/85 mm Hg.[42 43] These recommendations are based on studies in the general population[14]

Key messages

- This study showed that tight control of blood pressure based on captopril or atenolol as first agents and aiming for both a systolic blood pressure <150 mm Hg and diastolic pressure <85 mm Hg achieved a mean 144/82 mm Hg compared with 154/87 mm Hg in a control group

- 29% of patients in the tight control group required three or more hypotensive treatments

- Tight control of blood pressure reduced the risk of any non-fatal or fatal diabetic complications and of death related to diabetes; deterioration in visual acuity was also reduced

- Reducing blood pressure needs to have high priority in caring for patients with type 2 diabetes

and in patients with type 1 diabetes with microalbuminuria or established nephropathy.[18 19] Guidelines were formulated on the assumption that data relating to hypertensive non-diabetic subjects and relatively young patients with type 1 diabetes also applied to those with type 2 diabetes. The prevention of both macrovascular and microvascular disease observed in this study provides evidence for the necessity of tight blood pressure control in type 2 diabetes. The recommendations for the less strict "fair" or "acceptable" blood pressure control targets by some of the advisory groups of ≤160/95 mm Hg,[38] <160/90 mm Hg,[40 41] or <150/90 mm Hg[39] need to be reviewed in the light of the results of our study.

Conclusion

Hypertension is common in patients with type 2 diabetes, with a prevalence of 40-60% over the age range of 45 to 75. This study, embedded within the UK prospective diabetes study, shows that treatment with an angiotensin converting enzyme inhibitor or β blocker aiming for a blood pressure of <150/ 85 mm Hg substantially reduces the risk of death and complications due to diabetes. The management of blood pressure should have a high priority in the treatment of type 2 diabetes.

We appreciate the cooperation of the patients and many NHS and non-NHS staff at the centres. We thank Philip Bassett for editorial assistance, and Caroline Wood, Kathy Waring, and Lorraine Mallia for typing the manuscripts.

Contributors: Clinical centres of the hypertension in diabetes study: M R Stearne, S L Palmer, M S Hammersley, S L Franklin, R S Spivey, J C Levy, C R Tidy, N J Bell, J Steemson, B A Barrow, R Coster, K Waring, L Nolan, E Truscott, N Walravens, L Cook, H Lampard, C Merle, P Parker, J McVittie, I Draisey (Radcliffe Infirmary, Oxford); L E Murchison, A H E Brunt, M J Williams, D W Pearson, X M P Petrie, M E J Lean, D Walmsley, F Lyall, E Christie, J Church, E Thomson, A Farrow, J M Stowers, M Stowers, K McHardy, N Patterson (Royal Infirmary, Aberdeen); A D Wright, N A Levi, A C I Shearer, R J W Thompson, G Taylor, S Rayton, M Bradbury, A Glover, A Smyth-Osbourne, C Parkes, J Graham, P England, S Gyde, C Eagle, B Chakrabarti, J Smith, J Sherwell (Birmingham General Hospital); E M Kohner, A Dornhorst, M C Doddridge, M Dumskyj, S Walji, P Sharp, M Sleightholm, G Vanterpool, C Rose, G Frost, M Roseblade, S Elliott, S Forrester, M Foster, K Myers, R Chapman (Hammersmith Hospital, London); J R Hayes, R W Henry, M S Featherston, G P R Archbold, M Copeland, R Harper, I Richardson, S Martin, M Foster, H A Davison, (City Hospital, Belfast); D R Hadden, L Kennedy, A B Atkinson, A M Culbert, C Hegan, H Tennet, N Webb, I Robinson, J Holmes, M Foster, P M Bell, D R McCance, J Rutherford, S Nesbitt (Royal Victoria Hospital, Belfast); A S Spathis, S Hyer, M E Nanson, L M James, J M Tyrell, C Davis, P Strugnell, M Booth, H Petrie, D Clark, B Rice, S Hulland, J L Barron (St Helier Hospital, Carshalton); J S Yudkin, B J Gould, J Singer, A Badenock, S Walji, M Eckert, K Alibhai, E Marriot, C Cox, R Price, M Fernandez, A Ryle, S Clarke, G Wallace, E Mehmed, S MacFarlane (Whittington Hospital, London); R H Greenwood, J Wilson, M J Denholm, R C Temple, K Whitfield, F Johnson, C Munroe, S Gorick, E Duckworth, M Flatman, S Rainbow (Norfolk and Norwich Hospital, Norwich); L J Borthwick, D J Wheatcroft, R J Seaman, R A Christie, W Wheatcroft, P Musk, J White, S McDougal, M Bond, P Raniga (Lister Hospital, Stevenage); R W Newton, R T Jung, C Roxburgh, B Kilgallon, L Dick, M Foster, N Waugh, S Kilby, A Ellingford, J Burns (Ninewells Hospital, Dundee); C V Fox, M C Holloway, H M Coghill, N Hein, A Fox, W Cowan, M Richard, K Quested, S J Evans (Northampton Hospital); R B Paisey, N P R Brown, A J Tucker, R Paisey, F Garrett, J Hogg, P Park, K Williams, P Harvey, R Wilcocks, S Mason, J Frost, C Warren, P Rocket, L Bower (Torbay Hospital); J M Roland, D J Brown, J Youens, K Stanton-King, H Mungall, V Ball, W Maddison, D Donnelly, S King, P Griffin, S Smith, S Church, G Dunn, A Wilson, K Palmer (Peterborough General Hospital); P M Brown, D Humphriss, A J M Davidson, R Rose, L Armistead, S Townsend, P Poon (Scarborough Hospital); I D A Peacock, N J C Culverwell, M H Charlton, B P S Connolly, J Peacock, J Barrett, J Wain, W Beeston, G King, P G Hill (Derbyshire Royal Infirmary, Derby); A J M Boulton, A M Robertson, V Katoulis, A Olukoga, H McDonald, S Kumar, F Abouaesha, B Abuaisha, E A Knowles, S Higgins, J Booker, J Sunter, K Breislin, R Parker, P Raval, J Curwell, H Davenport, G Shawcross, A Prest, J Grey, H Cole, C Sereviratne (Manchester Royal Infirmary); R J Young, T L Dornan, J R Clyne, M Gibson, I O'Connell, L M Wong, S J Wilson, K L Wright, C Wallace, D McDowell (Hope Hospital, Salford); A C Burden, E M Sellen, R Gregory, M Roshan, N Vaghela, M Burden, C Sherriff, J Clarke, J Grenfell (Leicester General Hospital); J E Tooke, K MacLeod, C Searnark, M Rammell, C Pym, J Stockman, C Yeo, J Piper, L Leighton, E Green, M Hoyle, K Jones, A Hudson, A J James, A Shore, A Higham, B Martin (Royal Devon and Exeter Hospital, Exeter).

Coordinating centre: R C Turner, R R Holman (chief investigators); D R Matthews, H A W Neil (additional investigators); I M Stratton, C A Cull, H J McElroy, Z Mehta (statisticians); S E Manley (biochemist); V Frighi (research associate); R Peto (consultant statistician); A I Adler (epidemiologist); P A Bassett (administrator); D R Matthews (Oxford), A D Wright (Birmingham), T L Doman (Salford) (end point assessors); E M Kohner, S Aldington, H Lipinski, R Collum, K I Harrison, C Macintyre, S Skinner, A Mortemore, D Nelson, S Cockley, S Levien, L Bodsworth, R Willox, T Biggs, S Dove, E Beattie, M Gradwell, S Staples, R Lam, F Taylor, L Leung (retinal photography grading); M J Payne, R D Carter, S M Brownlee, K E Fisher, K Islam, R Jelfs, P A Williams, F A Williams, P J Sutton, A Ayres, L J Logie, M A Evans, L A Stowell (laboratory staff); E A Eeley (Oxford) (dietitian); I Ross (Aberdeen) (consultant biochemist); I A Kennedy (applications programmer); D Croft, E A Harris (database clerks); A H Keen, C Rose (Guy's Hospital) (electrocardiographic coding); M Raikou, A M Gray, A J McGuire, P Fenn (Oxford) (health economists); Z Mehta (Oxford), A E Fletcher, C Bulpitt, C Battersby (Hammersmith), J S Yudkin (Whittington) (quality of life questionnaire); R Stevens (Oxford) (mathematical modeller).

Previous participants: S F Oakes (administrator); J I Mann (epidemiologist); A Smith, Z Nugent (statisticians).

Committees: C A Cull, V Frighi, R R Holman, S E Manley, D R Matthews, H A W Neil, I M Stratton, R C Turner (United Kingdom prospective diabetes study data committee); W J H Butterfield, W R S Doll, R Eastman, F R Ferris, R R Holman, R Kurinij, R Peto, K McPherson, R F Mahler, T W Meade, G Shafer, R C Turner, P J Watkins, D Siegel (previous member) (Data monitoring and ethics committee). C V Fox, D R Hadden, R R Holman, D R Matthews, R C Turner, A D Wright, J S Yudkin (Policy Advisory Group). A B Atkinson, R R Holman, J G G Ledingham, L E Ramsay, R C Turner, A E G Raine (previous member) (Steering Committee for Hypertension in Diabetes Study). D J Betteridge, R D Cohen, D Currie, J Darbyshire, J V Forrester, T Guppy, R R Holman, D G Johnston, A McGuire, M Murphy, A M el-Nahas, B Pentecost, D Spiegelhalter, R C Turner (Medical Research Council and British Diabetic Association steering committee).

Guarantor: R C Turner.

Funding: The UK prospective diabetes study and the hypertension in diabetes study was funded by grants from the Medical Research Council, British Diabetic Association, Department of Health, the United States National Eye Institute and the United States National Institute of Diabetes, Digestive and Kidney Disease in the National Institutes of Health, the British Heart Foundation, the Charles Wolfson Charitable Trust, the Clothworkers' Foundation, the Health Promotion Research Trust, the Alan and Babette Sainsbury Trust, the Oxford University Medical Research Fund Committee, and pharmaceutical companies, including Novo-Nordisk, Bayer, Bristol-Myers Squibb, Hoechst, Lilly, Lipha, and Farmitalia Carlo Erba. GlaxoWellcome, Smith-Kline Beecham, Pfizer, Zeneca, Pharmacia and Upjohn, and Roche provided grants for health economics and epidemiological studies. Boehringer Mannheim, Becton Dickinson, Owen Mumford, Securicor, Kodak, and Cortecs Diagnostics gave additional help.

Conflict of interest: None.

1 Garcia MJ, McNamara PM, Gordon T, Kannell WB. Morbidity and mortality in diabetics in the Framingham population. Sixteen year follow-up. Diabetes 1974;23:105-11.
2 Stamler J, Vaccaro O, Neaton JD, Wentworth D. Diabetes, other risk factors, and 12 year cardiovascular mortality for men screened in the multiple risk factor intervention trial. Diabetes Care 1993;16:434-44.
3 Manson JAE, Colditz GA, Stampfer MJ, Willett WC, Krolewski AS, Rosner B, et al. A prospective study of maturity-onset diabetes mellitus and risk of coronary heart disease and stroke in women. Arch Intern Med 1991;151:1141-7.
4 Perneger TV, Brancati FL, Whelton PK, Klag MJ. End-stage renal disease attributable to diabetes mellitus. Ann Intern Med 1994;121:912-8.
5 Klag MJ, Whelton PK, Randall BL, Neaton JD, Brancati FL, Ford CE, et al. Blood pressure and end stage renal disease in men. N Engl J Med 1996;334:13-8.
6 United Kingdom Prospective Diabetes Study Group. UK Prospective Diabetes Study 23: risk factors for coronary artery disease in non-insulin dependent diabetes. BMJ 1998;316:823-8.
7 Hypertension in Diabetes Study Group. HDS 1: Prevalence of hypertension in newly presenting type 2 diabetic patients and the association with risk factors for cardio-vascular and diabetic complications. J Hypertens 1993;11:309-17.
8 Prescott-Clarke P, Primatesta P, eds. Health survey for England 1995. London: HMSO, 1997.
9 Harris MI, Cowie CC, Stern MP, Boyko EJ, Reiber GE, Bennett PH, eds. Diabetes in America. 2nd ed. Washington, DC: National Institutes of Health, National Institute of Diabetes and Digestive and Kidney Diseases, 1995.
10 Hypertension in Diabetes Study Group. HDS 2: Increased risk of cardio-vascular complications in hypertensive type 2 diabetic patients. J Hypertens 1993;11:319-25.
11 United Kingdom Prospective Diabetes Study Group. UK Prospective Diabetes Study X: urinary albumin excretion over 3 years in diet-treated type 2 (non-insulin-dependent) diabetic patients, and association with hypertension, hyperglycaemia and hypertriglyceridaemia. Diabetologia 1993;36:1021-9.
12 Nelson RG, Bennett PH, Beck GJ, Tan M, Knowler WC, Mitch WE, et al. Development and progression of renal disease in Pima Indians with non-insulin-dependent diabetes mellitus. N Engl J Med 1996;335:1636-42.
13 United Kingdom Prospective Diabetes Study Group. UK Prospective Diabetes Study 30: diabetic retinopathy at diagnosis of type 2 diabetes and associated risk factors. Arch Ophthalmol 1998;116:297-303.
14 Collins R, MacMahon S. Blood pressure, antihypertensive drug treatment and the risks of stroke and of coronary heart disease. Br Med Bull 1994;50:272-98.
15 Collins R, Peto R, MacMahon S, Herbert P, Fiebach NH, Eberlein KA, et al. Blood pressure, stroke, and coronary heart disease. Part 2. Short-term reductions in blood pressure: overview of randomised drug trials in their epidemiological context. Lancet 1990;335:827-38.
16 Medical Research Council Working Party. MRC trial of treatment of hypertension in older adults: principal results. BMJ 1992;304:405-12.
17 Sanderson S. Hypertension in the elderly: pressure to treat? Health Trends 1996;28:4:117-21.
18 Parving HH, Andersen M, Smidt UH, Hommel E, Mathiesen ER, Svendsen PA. Effect of antihypertensive treatment on kidney function in diabetic nephropathy. BMJ 1987;294:1443-7.
19 Mogensen C, Keane W, Bennett P, Jerums G, Parving H, Passa P, et al. Prevention of diabetic renal disease with special reference to microalbuminuria. Lancet 1995;346:1080-4.
20 Mogensen CE. Systemic blood pressure and glomerular leakage with particular reference to diabetes and hypertension. J Intern Med 1994;235:297-316.
21 Hypertension in Diabetes Study Group. HDS 3: Prospective study of therapy in type 2 diabetic patients—efficacy of ACE inhibitor and β-blocker. Diabet Med 1994;11:773-82.
22 United Kingdom Prospective Diabetes Study Group. UK prospective diabetes study VIII: study design, progress and performance. Diabetologia 1991;34:877-90.

71

23 United Kingdom Prospective Diabetes Study Group. UK prospective diabetes study 33: intensive blood glucose control with sulphonylureas or insulin compared with conventional treatment and risk of complications in patients with type 2 diabetes *Lancet* 1998;352:837-53.

24 British Diabetic Association. Dietary recommendations for diabetics for the 1980s. *Hum Nutr Appl Nutr* 1982;36:378-94.

25 Systolic Hypertension in the Elderly Program Cooperative Research Group. Prevention of stroke by antihypertensive drug treatment in older persons with isolated systolic hypertension. Final results of the systolic hypertension in the elderly program (SHEP). *JAMA* 1991;265:3255-64.

26 Dahlof B, Lindholm L, Hansson L, Scheriten B, Ekbom T, Wester PO. Morbidity and mortality in the Swedish trial in old patients with hypertension (STOP-Hypertension). *Lancet* 1991;338:1281-5.

27 United Kingdom Prospective Diabetes Study Group. UK Prospective Diabetes Study XI: biochemical risk factors in type 2 diabetic patients at diagnosis compared witn age-matched normal subjects. *Diabet Med* 1994;11:534-44.

28 Manley SE, Burton ME, Fisher KE, Cull CA, Tumer RC. Decreases in albumin/creatinine and N-acetylglucosaminidase/creatinine ratios in urine samples stored at −20°C. *Clin Chem* 1992;38:2294-9.

29 UK Prospective Diabetes Study Group. Efficacy of atenolol and captopril in reducing risk of macrovascular and microvascular complications in type 2 diabetes: UKPDS 39. *BMJ* 1998;317:713-20.

30 Curb JD, Pressel SL, Cutler JA, Savage P, Applegate WB, Black H, et al. Effect of diuretic-based antihypertensive treatment on cardiovascular disease risk in older diabetic patients with isolated systolic hypertension. Systolic Hypertension in the Elderly Program Cooperative Research Group. *JAMA* 1996;276:1886-92.

31 Hansson L, Zanchetti A, Carruthers SG, Dahlf B, Elmfeldt D, Julius S, et al. Effect of intensive blood-pressure lowering and low-dose aspirin in patients with hypertension: principal results of the hypertension optimal treatment (HOT) randomised trial. *Lancet* 1998;351:1755-62.

32 Hypertension Detection and Follow-up Program Cooperative Group. Mortality findings for stepped-care and referred-care participants in the Hypertension Detection and Follow-up Program, stratified by other risk factors. *Prev Med* 1985;14:312-35.

33 Klein R, Moss SE, Klein BE, Davis MD, DeMets DL. The Wisconsin Epidemiologic Study of Diabetic Retinopathy. XI. The incidence of macular edema. *Ophthalmology* 1989;96:1501-10.

34 Davies EG, Petty RG, Kohner EM. Long term effectiveness of photocoagulation for diabetic maculopathy. *Eye* 1989;3:764-7.

35 British Multicentre Group. Photocoagulation for proliferative diabetic retinopathy: a randomised controlled clinical trial using the xenon-arc. *Diabetologia* 1984;26:109-15.

36 Parving HH, Hommel E, Smidt UM. Protection of kidney function and decrease in albuminuria by captopril in insulin dependent diabetics with nephropathy. *BMJ* 1987;297:1086-91.

37 Ravid M, Savin H, Jutrin I, Bental T, Lang R, Lishner M. Long-term effect of ACE inhibition on development of nephropathy in diabetes mellitus type II. *Kidney Int* 1994;45(suppl):S161-4.

38 Alberti KGMM, Gries FA, Jervell J, Krans HM. A desktop guide for the management of non-insulin-dependent diabetes mellitus (NIDDM): an update. *Diabetic Med* 1994;11:899-909.

39 Canadian Diabetes Advisory Board. Clinical practice guidelines. *Can Med Assoc J* 1992;147:697-712.

40 Bauduceau B, Chatellier G, Cordonnier D, Marre M, Mimran A, Monnier L, et al. Hypertension arterielle et diabète. Membres des conseils d'administration et scientifiques de l'ALFEDIAM. *Diabetes Metab* 1996;22:64-76.

41 RR Associates. *Blood pressure and diabetes: everyone's concern*. London: British Diabetic Association, 1994.

42 American Diabetes Association. Standards of medical care for patients with diabetes mellitus. *Diabetes Care* 1998;21(suppl):S23-31.

43 Joint National Committee on Prevention, Detection, Evaluation and Treatment of High Blood Pressure. Sixth report. *Arch Intern Med* 1997;157:2413-46.

(Accepted 17 August 1998)

The unpredictability paradox: review of empirical comparisons of randomised and non-randomised clinical trials

Regina Kunz, Andrew D Oxman

Abstract

Objective To summarise comparisons of randomised clinical trials and non-randomised clinical trials, trials with adequately concealed random allocation versus inadequately concealed random allocation, and high quality trials versus low quality trials where the effect of randomisation could not be separated from the effects of other methodological manoeuvres.

Design Systematic review.

Selection criteria Cohorts or meta-analyses of clinical trials that included an empirical assessment of the relation between randomisation and estimates of effect.

Data sources Cochrane Review Methodology Database, Medline, SciSearch, bibliographies, hand searching of journals, personal communication with methodologists, and the reference lists of relevant articles.

Main outcome measures Relation between randomisation and estimates of effect.

Results Eleven studies that compared randomised controlled trials with non-randomised controlled trials (eight for evaluations of the same intervention and three across different interventions), two studies that compared trials with adequately concealed random allocation and inadequately concealed random allocation, and five studies that assessed the relation between quality scores and estimates of treatment effects, were identified. Failure to use random allocation and concealment of allocation were associated with relative increases in estimates of effects of 150% or more, relative decreases of up to 90%, inversion of the estimated effect and, in some cases, no difference. On average, failure to use randomisation or adequate concealment of allocation resulted in larger estimates of effect due to a poorer prognosis in non-randomly selected control groups compared with randomly selected control groups.

Conclusions Failure to use adequately concealed random allocation can distort the apparent effects of care in either direction, causing the effects to seem either larger or smaller than they really are. The size of these distortions can be as large as or larger than the size of the effects that are to be detected.

Introduction

> Observational evidence is clearly better than opinion, but it is thoroughly unsatisfactory. All research on the effectiveness of therapy was in this unfortunate state until the early 1950s. The only exceptions were the drugs whose effect on immediate mortality were so obvious that no trials were necessary, such as insulin, sulphonamide, and penicillin.[1]

"The basic idea, like most good things, is very simple."[1] Randomisation is the only means of controlling for unknown and unmeasured differences between comparison groups as well as those that are known and measured. Random assignment removes the potential of bias in the assignment of patients to one intervention or another by introducing unpredictability. When alternation or any other preset plan (such as time of admission) is used, it is possible to arrange to enter a patient into a study at an opportune moment. With randomisation, however, each patient's treatment is assigned according to the play of chance. It is a paradox that unpredictability is introduced into the design of clinical trials by using random allocation to protect against the unpredictability of the extent of bias in the results of non-randomised clinical trials.

Despite this simple logic, and many examples of harm being done because of delays in conducting randomised trials, there are limitations to the use of randomised trials, both real and imagined, and scepticism about the value of randomisation.[2-5] We believe this scepticism is healthy. It is important to question assumptions about research methods, and to test these assumptions empirically, just as it is important to test assumptions about the effects of health care. In this paper we have attempted systematically to summarise empirical studies of the relation between randomisation and estimates of effect.

Methods

We included four types of comparisons in our review: randomised clinical trials versus non-randomised clinical trials of the same intervention, randomised clinical trials versus non-randomised clinical trials across different interventions, adequately concealed random allocation versus inadequately concealed random allocation in trials, and high quality trials versus low quality trials in which the specific effect of randomisation or allocation concealment could not be separated from the effect of other methodological manoeuvres such as double blinding. Both descriptive and analytical assessments of the relation between the use of random allocation and estimates of effect are included, based on cohorts or meta-analyses of clinical trials.

We identified studies from the Cochrane Review Methodology Database,[6] other methodological bibliographies, Medline, and SciSearch, and by hand searching journals, personal communication with methodologists, and checking the reference lists of relevant articles. These searches were conducted up to July 1998. Potentially relevant citations were retrieved and assessed for inclusion independently by both authors. Disagreements were resolved by discussion.

We used the following criteria to appraise the methodological quality of included studies: Were explicit criteria used to select the trials? Did two or more investigators agree regarding the selection of

Department of Nephrology, Charité, Berlin, Germany
Regina Kunz, *registrar*

Health Services Research Unit, National Institute of Public Health, Oslo, Norway
Andrew D Oxman, *director*

Correspondence to:
Dr Oxman
andrew.oxman@labmed.uio.no

BMJ 1998;317:1185–90

Originally published in *BMJ* 1998; **317**: 1185–90.

trials? Was there a consecutive or complete sample of clinical trials? Did the study control for other methodological differences such as double blinding and complete follow up? Did the study control for clinical differences in the participants and interventions in the included trials? Were similar outcome measures used in the included trials? The overall quality of each study was summarised as: no important flaws, possibly important flaws, or major flaws.

For each study one of us (RK) extracted information about the sample of clinical trials, the comparison that was made, the type of analysis undertaken, and the results, and the other checked the extracted data against the published article. The reported relation between randomisation and estimates of effect was recorded and, if possible, converted to the relative overestimation or underestimation of the relative risk reduction. We prepared tables for each type of comparison to facilitate a qualitative analysis of the extent to which the included studies yielded similar results, and heterogeneity in the included studies was explored both within and across comparisons.

In summarising the results we have assumed that evidence from randomised trials is the reference standard to which estimates from non-randomised trials are compared. However, as with other gold standards, randomised trials are not without flaws, and this assumption is not intended to imply that the true effect is known, or that estimates derived from randomised trials are always closer to the truth than estimates from non-randomised trials.

Results

We have identified 18 cohorts or meta-analyses that met our inclusion criteria, totalling 1211 clinical trials.[7-24] Efforts to develop an efficient electronic search strategy using Medline have thus far not been successful due to poor indexing. Searches for studies that cited Colditz and colleagues,[15] Miller and colleagues,[16] Chalmers and colleagues,[18] or Schulz and colleagues[19] using SciSearch yielded seven additional studies. Searches using SciSearch for studies that cited the other studies meeting our inclusion criteria did not yield any other additional studies. Exploratory hand searching of three methodological journals (*Controlled Clinical Trials*, *Statistics in Medicine*, and the *Journal of Clinical Epidemiology*) for four years (1970, 1980, 1990, and 1995) yielded a single relevant study published in 1990. The 18 included studies were published in 14 different journals. The majority of studies were identified through personal communication with methodologists and through bibliographies and reference lists.

Table 1 Randomised controlled trials (RCTs) compared with non-randomised controlled trials (non-RCTs) of the same intervention

Study	Sample (search strategy)	Comparison	Results	Direction of bias
Chalmers 1977[7]	32 controlled studies of anticoagulation in acute myocardial infarction (systematic)	RCTs with CCTs and HCTs on case fatality rate, rate of thromboembolism, and haemorrhages	Relative risk reduction for mortality overestimated by 35% in HCTs and 6% in CCTs compared with RCTs. Case fatality rate highest in HCTs (38.3%) compared with RCTs (19.6%) and CCTs (29.2%). Similar pattern for thromboembolism	Overestimation of effect
Sacks 1982[8]	Sample of 50 RCTs and 56 HCTs, assessing 6 interventions (treatment of oesophageal varices, coronary artery surgery, anticoagulation in myocardial infarction, chemotherapy for colon cancer and melanoma, and diethylstilboestrol for recurrent miscarriage) (at hand)	RCTs with HCTs on frequency of detecting statistically significant results ($P \leq 0.05$) of primary outcome and reduction of mortality	20% of the RCTs found a statistically significant benefit from the new treatment compared with 79% of the HCTs. Relative risk reduction of mortality in HCTs v RCTs was 0.49/0.27 (1.8) for cirrhosis, 0.68/0.26 (2.6) for coronary artery surgery at 3 years, 0.49/0.22 (2.2) for anticoagulation in myocardial infarction, and 0.67/−0.02 for diethylstilboestrol in recurrent miscarriage. Outcomes in treatment groups were similar in both designs, but outcomes in control groups were worse among historical controls	Overestimation of effect
Diehl 1986[9]	19 RCTs and 17 HCTs for 6 types of cancer (breast, colon, stomach, lung cancer, melanoma, soft tissue sarcoma) (reference lists of two textbooks)	Matching of randomised and historical controls for disease, stage, and follow up, and comparison on survival and relapse free survival	18 of 43 matched control groups (42%) varied by >10% (absolute difference in either outcome), 9 (21%) by >20%, and 2 (5%) by >30%. Survival or relapse free survival was better in RCTs compared with HCTs in 17/18 matches	Overestimation of effect
Reimold 1992[10]	6 RCTs and 6 CCTs of chinidine in atrial fibrillation (systematic)	RCTs and CCTs on maintenance of sinus rhythm 3, 6, and 12 months after cardioversion	At 3 months, beneficial effect of maintaining sinus rhythm with chinidine was 54% less in non-RCTs compared with RCTs, and was 76% less at 12 months	Underestimation of effect
Recurrent Miscarriage Immunotherapy Trialists Group 1994[11]	9 RCTs and 6 CCTs (with self selected treatment) of allogenic leucocyte immunotherapy for recurrent miscarriage (systematic)	RCTs and CCTs on live birth rate	Beneficial effect of immunotherapy on birth rate among pregnant women was 9% larger in CCTs compared with RCTs, but was 63% lower in CCTs when all women were considered	Underestimation of effect when all women considered, similar effect for pregnant women
Watson 1994[12]	4 RCTs and 6 CCTs/HCTs of oil soluble contrast media during hysterosalpingography in infertile couples (systematic)	RCTs and CCTs/HCTs on pregnancy rate	RCTs and CCTs/HCTs detected similar increases in pregnancy rates: odds ratio for RCTs 1.92 (95% CI, 1.33 to 2.68) and for CCTs/HCTs 1.92 (1.55 to 2.38)	Similar effect
Pyörälä 1995[13]	11 RCTs and 22 (not further specified) non-RCTs on hormonal therapy in cryptorchidism (systematic)	RCTs and non-RCTs on the descent of testes after therapy with luteinising hormone releasing hormone or human chorionic gonadotrophin	Success rate of descent of testes after therapy with luteinising hormone releasing hormone was 2.3 times larger in non-RCTs than in RCTs and 1.7 times larger after therapy with human chorionic gonadotrophin	Overestimation of effect
Carroll 1996[14]	17 RCTs and 19 non-RCTs (including HCTs or trials with inadequate randomisation procedures) on transcutaneous electrical nerve stimulation (systematic)	RCTs and non-RCTs on control of postoperative pain	Transcutaneous electrical nerve stimulation judged ineffective at improving postoperative pain in 85% of RCTs, while 89% of non-RCTs concluded that it did improve postoperative pain	Overestimation of effect

CCT=concurrently controlled trial; HCT=historically controlled trial.

Table 2 Randomised controlled trials (RCTs) compared with non-randomised controlled trials (non-RCTs) across different interventions

Study	Sample (search strategy)	Comparison	Results	Direction of bias
Colditz 1989[15]	113 studies published in 1980 comparing new interventions with old, identified in leading cardiology, neurology, psychiatry, and respiratory journals (systematic)	36 parallel RCTs, 29 randomised COTs, 46 non-randomised COTs, 3 CCTs, 5 ECTs, 9 observational studies compared for "treatment gain" (Mann-Whitney statistic), and relation between quality score and "treatment gain" assessed	All but one design achieved similar "treatment gains" (0.56-0.65). Overall, 89% of new treatments were rated as improvements, but only non-randomised COTs detected a significantly higher "treatment gain" from the new treatment compared with RCTs (P=0.004). Within RCTs, there was no correlation between quality score and "treatment gain" (P=0.18)	Inconclusive
Miller 1989[16]	188 studies comparing new surgical interventions with old, published in 1983 and identified in leading surgical journals (systematic)	81 RCTs, 15 CCTs, 27 HCTs, 91 observational studies, 7 BASs compared on "treatment gain" (Mann-Whitney), and association between treatment success and study design and the relation between quality score and treatment gains assessed	Non-significant trend towards larger "treatment gains" for new treatments on the principal disease in non-RCTs (0.56 to 0.78) than in RCTs (0.56). For treatment of complications the "treatment gain" was similar across all study designs (0.54 to 0.55) except in BASs (0.90). Within RCTs, there was no correlation between quality scores and treatment gains (P=0.7)	Inconclusive
Ottenbacher 1992[17]	Sample of 30 RCTs and 30 trials with non-random process of allocation, eg matching or HCTs (systematic search of *N Engl J Med* and *JAMA* across several medical specialties)	RCTs and non-RCTs on treatment effects as measured by standardised mean differences	No difference in treatment effect found between non-RCTs (0.23) and RCTs (0.21)	Similar effects

COT=Crossover trial; CCT=concurrently controlled trial; ECT=external control study; BAS=before and after study; HCT=historically controlled trial.

Randomised trials versus non-randomised trials of the same intervention

Table 1 summarises the eight studies comparing randomised clinical trials and non-randomised clinical trials of the same intervention. In five of the eight studies, estimates of effect were larger in non-randomised trials. Outcomes in the randomised treatment groups and non-randomised treatment groups were frequently similar, but worse outcomes among historical controls spuriously increased the estimated treatment effects. One study found comparable results for both allocation procedures, and two studies reported smaller treatment effects in non-randomised studies. In one study the smaller estimate of effect was due to a poorer prognosis for patients in the non-randomised treatment groups. The deviation of the estimates of effect for non-randomised trials compared with randomised trials ranged from an underestimation of effect of 76% to an overestimation of effect of 160%.

Randomised trials versus non-randomised trials across different interventions

The evidence from comparisons across different interventions and various study designs (randomised controlled trials and non-randomised controlled trials, crossover designs, and observational studies) is less clear (table 2). In all three studies several study designs and clinical conditions were combined and their diverse outcomes converted to a standardised effect size. There was substantial clinical heterogeneity, and there were many other factors that could distort or mask a possible association between randomisation and estimates of effect. No consistent relation between study design or quality and the magnitude of the estimates of effect was detected.

Adequately concealed allocation versus inadequately concealed allocation

Concealed random allocation to treatment—that is, blinding of the randomisation schedule to prevent subversion by the investigators or trial participants—should ensure protection against biased allocation. Chalmers and colleagues found that within randomised controlled trials failure adequately to conceal allocation was associated with larger imbalances in prognostic factors and larger treatment effects (table 3).[18] They reported a more than sevenfold overestimation of the treatment effect in trials with inadequately concealed allocation. They did not, however, control for other methodological factors in their descriptive analysis.[18] Schulz and colleagues conducted a multivariate analysis that controlled for blinding and completeness of follow up, which yielded similar results.[19] They found that inadequately concealed random allocation (for example, alternation) compared with adequately concealed random allocation (for example, assignment by a central office) resulted in

Table 3 Trials with adequately concealed allocation compared with inadequately concealed allocation

Study	Sample (search strategy)	Comparison	Results	Direction of bias
Chalmers 1983[18]	145 controlled trials of treatment for acute myocardial infarction (systematic)	Studies with different allocation schemes (non-random, non-concealed random, and concealed random allocation) on maldistribution of prognostic variables, frequency of significant outcomes, and case fatality rates	In non-RCTs, non-concealed RCTs, and RCTs with concealed allocation, the maldistribution of prognostic factors was 34%, 7%, and 3.5% respectively, frequency of significant outcomes was 25%, 11%, and 5% respectively, average relative risk reduction for mortality was 33%, 23%, and 3% respectively. Case fatality rate for control groups was 32%, 23%, and 16% and for treatment groups was 21%, 18%, and 16% respectively	Overestimation of effect
Schulz 1995[19]	250 RCTs from 33 meta-analyses (Cochrane Pregnancy and Childbirth Database)	Association between methodological features of controlled trials (allocation concealment, double blinding, and follow up), and treatment effect (odds ratio)	Treatment effect overestimated by 41% in RCTs with inadequate concealment and by 30% in RCTs with unclear adequacy of concealment compared with those with adequate concealment (P≤0.001) after adjustment for other methodological features. Studies with no double blinding overestimated treatment effect by 17% compared with double blinded studies (P =0.01). Lack of complete follow up had no influence on treatment effect (7%, P=0.32)	Overestimation of effect

RCT=Randomised controlled trial.

Table 4 Studies of high quality trials compared with low quality trials

Study	Sample (search strategy)	Comparison	Results	Direction of bias
Emerson 1990[20]	Sample of 7 meta-analyses with 107 primary studies where full information about quality scores was available (at hand)	Assessment of relation between quality score and (a) observed treatment difference and (b) variation of observed treatment difference	No correlation detected between either quality score and treatment difference or variation of treatment difference within each meta-analysis or in combined analysis (P=0.29)	Similar effects
Imperiale 1990[21]	Meta-analysis of 11 RCTs of steroids in alcoholic hepatitis (systematic)	Short term mortality in studies with high and low methodological quality	In studies with low quality, relative risk reduction on mortality was 86% smaller than the reduction observed in high quality studies. In studies with low quality and hepatic encephalopathy no effect was observed, while the relative risk reduction of mortality in high quality studies was 55%	Underestimation of effect
Nurmohamed 1992[22]	Meta-analysis of 35 surgical and orthopaedic RCTs on low molecular weight heparin as thromboprophylaxis (systematic)	Relative risk reduction for deep vein thrombosis and pulmonary embolism in studies of high and low methodological quality	In studies with low quality, relative risk reduction for venous thrombosis in surgical trials was 2.6 times larger, and in orthopaedic trials 1.4 times larger, than studies with high quality. Relative risk reduction for pulmonary embolus in surgical trials was 1.7 times larger, and in orthopaedic trials 2.8 times larger, than studies with high quality	Overestimation of effect
Khan 1996[23]	Meta-analysis of 9 RCTs (parallel or crossover design) evaluating the effect of anti-oestrogen treatment in male infertility (systematic)	Pregancy rates in studies with high and low methodological quality	In studies of low quality, pregnancy rate increased under treatment (odds ratio 2.6), but declined under treatment in high quality studies (0.5)	Reversal of effect
Ortiz 1998[24]	Meta-analysis of 7 RCTs on the effect of folic or folinic acid v placebo (systematic)	Frequency of gastrointestinal side effects in studies with high and low methodological quality	In studies with low quality there was a 43% reduction in the odds ratio of side effects (0.57) compared with a 70% reduction in studies with high quality (0.3)	Underestimation of effect

RCT=Randomised controlled trial.

estimates of effect (odds ratios) that were on average 40% larger.

High quality trials versus low quality trials

Considerable differences in the observed treatment effect were detected when the results of high quality studies were compared with those of low quality studies in the context of systematic reviews of specific health care (table 4). In these studies the estimates of effect were distorted in both directions and even caused the alarming situation of a harmful intervention associated with a reduction in pregnancies (odds ratio 0.5, on the basis of high quality studies) seeming beneficial in low quality studies (odds ratio 2.6, on the basis of low quality studies). In two meta-analyses, low quality studies consistently underestimated the beneficial effect of the intervention being evaluated by 27% to 100%, and an effective treatment could have been discarded based on the results of low quality studies.

Methodological quality

The methodological quality of the studies included in this review varied. Four studies met all of our criteria.[19 21–23] Three of these assessed the impact of bias on the effect of a specific healthcare intervention as part of a systematic review, and the analysis was performed as part of a subgroup analysis to test the robustness of the overall finding.[21–23] The other 14 studies had one or more methodological flaws including not controlling for other methodological manoeuvres[16 18 22 27] or clinical differences.[7 13–17 20 24]

Discussion

It has proved difficult to develop efficient search strategies for locating empirical methodological studies such as the ones included in this review. Although we believe it is unlikely that there are many published methodological studies such as the ones by Sacks and colleagues,[8] Schulz and colleagues,[19] Chalmers and colleagues,[18] and Emerson and colleagues[20] that we have not identified, there may be unpublished

or ongoing studies like these that we have not identified, and it is likely that there are many meta-analyses that meet the inclusion criteria for this review that we have not identified. The Cochrane Library contains 428 completed reviews and 397 protocols, and there are over 1700 entries in the database of abstracts of reviews of effectiveness.[26] We have not systematically gone through all of these meta-analyses. An expanded version of this review will be published in the Cochrane Library and kept up to date through the Cochrane Empirical Methodological Studies Methods Group.[27] Additional studies will be added to the review, and any errors that are identified will be corrected.

We have not included comparisons between randomised controlled trials and cohort studies,[28] case-control studies,[29 30] or evaluations of effectiveness using large healthcare administrative databases,[3] although some of the studies in this review included observational studies. Observational studies often provide valuable information that is complementary to the results of clinical trials. For example, case-control studies may be the best available study design for evaluating rare adverse effects, and large database studies may provide important information about the extent to which effects that are expected based on randomised clinical trials are achieved in routine practice. However, it is important to remember that it is only possible to control for confounders that are known and measured in observational studies, and we should be wary of hubris and its consequences in assuming that we know all there is to know about any disease.

As with any review the quality of the data is limited by the quality of the studies that we have reviewed. Most of the studies included in the review had one or more methodological flaws. In many of the included comparisons, particularly those between randomised controlled trials and historically controlled trials, methodological differences other than randomisation may account for some of the observed differences in estimates of effect.[7–9 13 18]

Four of the studies met all of our criteria for assessing methodological quality,[19 21–23] and one study in particular provided strong support for the conclusion that clinical trials that lack adequately concealed random allocation produce estimates of effect that are on average 40% larger than clinical trials with adequately concealed random allocation, but that the degree and the direction of this bias varies widely.[19] This study also shows the potential contribution that systematic reviews, and notably the Cochrane Database of Systematic Reviews, can make towards developing an empirical basis for methodological decisions in evaluations of health care. Currently this empirical basis is lacking, and many methodological debates rely more on logic or rhetoric than evidence. Analyses such as the one undertaken by Schulz and colleagues, in which methodological comparisons are made among trials of the same intervention, are likely to yield more reliable results than comparisons that are made across different interventions which, not surprisingly, tend to be inconclusive.[15–17]

We have assumed that, in general, differences between randomised trials and non-randomised trials or between trials with adequately concealed random allocation and inadequately concealed random allocation are best explained by bias in the non-randomised controlled trials and inadequately concealed trials. This assumption is supported by findings of large imbalances in prognostic factors as well. However, it is possible that randomised controlled trials can sometimes underestimate the effectiveness of an intervention in routine practice by forcing healthcare professionals and patients to acknowledge their uncertainty and thereby reduce the strength of placebo effects.[4 25 31] It is also possible that publication bias can partly explain some of the differences in results observed in studies such as the one by Sacks and colleagues.[8] This would be the case if randomised trials are more likely to be published regardless of the effect size, than historically controlled trials. However, we are not aware of any evidence that supports this hypothesis, and the available evidence shows consistently that randomised trials, like other research, are also more likely to be published if they have results that are considered significant.[32–35]

Several explanations for discrepancies between estimates of effect derived from randomised trials and non-randomised trials are possible. For example, it can be argued that estimates of effect might be larger in randomised trials if the care provided in the context of trials is better than that in routine practice, assuming this is the case for the treatment group and not the control group. Similarly, strict eligibility criteria might select people with a higher capacity to benefit from a treatment, resulting in larger estimates of effect in randomised trials than non-randomised trials with less strict eligibility criteria. If, for some reason, patients with a poor prognosis were more likely to be allocated to the treatment group in non-randomised trials then this would also result in larger estimates of effect in randomised trials. Conversely, if patients with a poor prognosis were more likely to be allocated to the control group in non-randomised trials, as often seems to be the case based on the results of this review, this would result in larger estimates of effect in the non-randomised trials.

> **Key messages**
>
> - Empirical studies support using random allocation in clinical trials and ensuring that the allocation process is concealed—that is, that assignment is impervious to any influence by the people making the allocation
>
> - The effect of not using concealed random allocation can be as large or larger than the effects of worthwhile interventions
>
> - On average, failure to use concealed random allocation results in overestimates of effect due to a poorer prognosis in non-randomly selected control groups compared with randomly selected control groups, but it can result in underestimates of effect, reverse the direction of effect, mask an effect, or give similar estimates of effect
>
> - The adequacy of allocation concealment may be a more sensitive measure of bias in clinical trials than scales used to assess the quality of clinical trials
>
> - It is a paradox that the unpredictability of randomisation is the best protection against the unpredictability of the extent and direction of bias in clinical trials that are not properly randomised

Conclusion

Overall, this review supports using random allocation in clinical trials and ensuring that the randomisation schedule is adequately concealed. The effect of not using random allocation with adequate concealment can be as large or larger than the effects of worthwhile interventions. On average, non-randomised trials and randomised trials with inadequately concealed allocation result in overestimates of effect. This bias, however, can go in either direction, can reverse the direction of effect, or can mask an effect.

For those undertaking clinical trials this review provides support for using randomisation to assemble comparison groups.[25] For those undertaking systematic reviews of clinical trials, this review provides support for considering sensitivity analyses based on the adequacy of allocation concealment in addition to or instead of on the basis of overall quality scores, which may be less sensitive measures of bias.

As Cochrane stated: "The [randomised controlled trial] is a very beautiful technique, of wide applicability, but as with everything else there are snags."[1] Those making decisions on the basis of clinical trials need to be cautious of small trials (even when they are properly randomised) and systematic reviews of small trials both because of chance effects and the risk of biased reporting.[36 37] It is also possible to introduce bias into a trial despite allocation concealment.[19 38] Finally, even when the risk of error due to either bias or chance is small, judgments must be made about the applicability of the results to individual patients[39 40] and about the relative value of the probable benefits, harms, and costs.[41 42]

We thank Alex Jadad, Steve Halpern, and David Cowan for help in locating studies, Dave Sackett and Iain Chalmers for encouragement and advice, Mike Clarke for reviewing the manuscript,

Annie Britton and other colleagues for provision of their bibliographies on research methodology, and the investigators who conducted the studies we reviewed.

Contributors: RK and ADO contributed to the preparation of the protocol and the final manuscript and assessed the relevance and methodological quality of retrieved reports. RK prepared the first drafts of the protocol and the paper, undertook the majority of the searches with help from David Cowan, Steve Halpern, Alex Jadad, and collected data from the included studies. ADO checked the collected data against the original reports. Both authors will act as guarantors for the paper.

Funding: Norwegian Ministry of Health and Social Affairs.
Competing interests: None declared.

1 Cochrane AL. *Effectiveness and efficiency: random reflections on health services.* London: Nuffield Provincial Hospitals Trust, 1972:20-5.
2 Committee for Evaluating Medical Technologies in Clinical Use. *Assessing medical technologies.* Washington DC: National Academy Press, 1985:76-8.
3 US Congress, Office of Technology Assessment. *Identifying health technologies that work: searching for evidence,* OTA-H-608. Washington DC: US Government Printing Office, 1994:41-51.
4 Black N. Why we need observational studies to evaluate the effectiveness of health care. *BMJ* 1996;312:1215-8.
5 Weiss CH. Evaluation. *Methods for studying programs and policies.* 2nd ed. Upper Saddle River: Prentice Hall, 1998:229-33.
6 Clarke M, Carling C, Oxman AD, eds. Cochrane Review Methodology Database. *The Cochrane Library.* Oxford: Update Software, 1998. Issue 3.
7 Chalmers TC, Matta RJ, Smith H Jr, Kunzler AM. Evidence favoring the use of anticoagulants in the hospital phase of acute myocardial infarction. *N Engl J Med* 1977;297:1091-6.
8 Sacks H, Chalmers TC, Smith H Jr. Randomized versus historical controls for clinical trials. *Am J Med* 1982;72:233-40.
9 Diehl LF, Perry DJ. A comparison of randomized concurrent control groups with matched historical control groups: are historical controls valid? *J Clin Oncol* 1986;4:1114-20.
10 Reimold SC, Chalmers TC, Berlin JA, Antman EM. Assessment of the efficacy and safety of antiarrhythmic therapy for chronic atrial fibrillation: observations on the role of trial design and implications of drug related mortality. *Am Heart J* 1992;124:924-32.
11 Recurrent Miscarriage Immunotherapy Trialists Group. Worldwide collaborative observational study and meta analysis on allogenic leukocyte immunotherapy for recurrent spontaneous abortion. *Am J Reprod Immunol* 1994;32:55-72.
12 Watson A, Vandekerckhove P, Lilford R, Vail A, Brosens I, Hughes E. A meta-analysis of the therapeutic role of oil soluble contrast media at hysterosalpingography: a surprising result? *Fertil Steril* 1994;61:470-7.
13 Pyorala S, Huttunen NP, Uhari M. A review and meta-analysis of hormonal treatment of cryptorchidism. *J Clin Endocrinol Metab* 1995;80:2795-9.
14 Carroll D, Tramer M, McQuay H, Nye B, Moore A. Randomization is important in studies with pain outcomes: systematic review of transcutaneous electrical nerve stimulation in acute postoperative pain. *Br J Anaesth* 1996;77:798-803.
15 Colditz GA, Miller JN, Mosteller F. How study design affects outcomes in comparisons of therapy. I: medical. *Stat Med* 1989;8:441-54.
16 Miller JN, Colditz GA, Mosteller F. How study design affects outcomes in comparisons of therapy. II: surgical. *Stat Med* 1989;8:455-66.
17 Ottenbacher K. Impact of random assignment on study outcome: an empirical examination. *Control Clin Trials* 1992;13:50-61.
18 Chalmers TC, Celano P, Sacks HS, Smith H Jr. Bias in treatment assignment in controlled clinical trials. *N Engl J Med* 1983;309:1358-61.
19 Schulz KF, Chalmers I, Hayes RJ, Altman DG. Empirical evidence of bias. Dimensions of methodological quality associated with estimates of treatment effects in controlled trials. *JAMA* 1995;273:408-12.
20 Emerson JD, Burdick E, Hoaglin DC, Mosteller F, Chalmers TC. An empirical study of the possible relation of treatment differences to quality scores in controlled randomized clinical trials. *Control Clin Trials* 1990;11:339-52.

21 Imperiale TF, McCullough AJ. Do corticosteroids reduce mortality from alcoholic hepatitis? A meta analysis of the randomized trials. *Ann Intern Med* 1990;113:299-307.
22 Nurmohamed MT, Rosendaal FR, Buller HR, Dekker E, Hommes DW, Vandenbroucke JP, et al. Low molecular weight heparin versus standard heparin in general and orthopaedic surgery: a meta-analysis. *Lancet* 1992;340:152-6.
23 Khan KS, Daya S, Jadad A. The importance of quality of primary studies in producing unbiased systematic reviews. *Arch Intern Med* 1996;156:661-6.
24 Ortiz Z, Shea B, Suarez Almazor ME, Moher D, Wells GA, Tugwell P. The efficacy of folic acid and folinic acid in reducing methotrexate gastrointestinal toxicity in rheumatoid arthritis. A meta-analysis of randomized controlled trials. *J Rheumatol* 1998;25:36-43.
25 Chalmers I. Assembling comparison groups to assess the effects of health care. *J R Soc Med* 1997;90:379-86.
26 NHS Centre for Reviews and Dissemination. Database of abstracts of reviews of effectiveness. *The Cochrane Library.* Oxford: Update Software, 1998. Issue 3.
27 Cochrane Empirical Methodological Studies Methods Group. *The Cochrane Library.* Oxford: Update Software, 1998. Issue 3.
28 Forgie MA, Wells PS, Laupacis A, Fergusson D. Preoperative autologous donation decreases allogeneic transfusion but increases exposure to all red blood cell transfusion: results of a meta-analysis. *Arch Intern Med* 1998;158:610-6.
29 Colditz GA, Brewer TF, Berkey CS, Wilson ME, Burdick E, Fineberg HV, et al. Efficacy of BCG vaccine in the prevention of tuberculosis. Meta analysis of the published literature. *JAMA* 1994;271:698-702.
30 Stieb D, Frayha HH, Oxman AD, Shannon HS, Hutchison BG, Crombie F. The effectiveness and usefulness of Haemophilus influenzae type b vaccines: a systematic overview (meta-analysis). *Can Med Assoc J* 1990;142:719-32.
31 Kleijnen J, Gøtzsche P, Kunz RH, Oxman AD, Chalmers I. So what's so special about randomisation? In: Maynard A, Chalmers I, eds. *Non-random reflections on health services research: on the 25th anniversary of Archie Cochrane's effectiveness and efficiency.* London: BMJ Publishing Group, 1997:93-106.
32 Dickersin K, Min YI. NIH clinical trials and publication bias. *Online J Curr Clin Trials* [serial online] 1993; document No 50.
33 Dickersin K. How important is publication bias? A synthesis of available data. *AIDS Education and Prevention* 1997;9(suppl A):15-21.
34 Stern JM, Simes RJ. Publication bias: evidence of delayed publication of clinical research projects. *BMJ* 1997;315:640-5.
35 Ioannidis JPA. Effect of the statistical significance of results on the time to completion and publication of randomized efficacy trials. *JAMA* 1998;279:281-6.
36 Counsell CE, Clarke MJ, Slattery J, Sandercock PAG. The miracle of DICE therapy for acute stroke: fact or fictional product of subgroup analysis? *BMJ* 1994;309:1677-81.
37 Egger M, Davey SG, Schneider M, Minder C. Bias in meta-analysis detected by a simple, graphical test. *BMJ* 1997;315:629-34.
38 Guyatt GH, Sackett DL, Cook DJ, for the Evidence-Based Working Group. Users' guides to the medical literature, II: how to use an article about therapy or prevention, A: are the results of the study valid? *JAMA* 1993;270:2598-601.
39 Dans AL, Dans LF, Guyatt GH, Richardson S. Users' guides to the medical literature: XIV. How to decide on the applicability of clinical trial results to your patient. *JAMA* 1998;279:545-9.
40 Cochrane Methods Working Group on Applicability and Recommendations. *The Cochrane Library.* Oxford: Update Software, 1998. Issue 3.
41 Guyatt GH, Sackett DL, Cook DJ, for the Evidence-Based Working Group. Users' guides to the medical literature, II: how to use an article about therapy or prevention, B: what were the results and will they help me in caring for my patients? *JAMA* 1994;270:59-63.
42 Oxman AD, Flottorp S. An overview of strategies to promote implementation of evidence based health care. In: Silagy C, Haines A, eds. *Evidence based practice.* London: BMJ Books, 1998:91-109.

(Accepted 29 September 1998)

Numbers needed to treat, odds ratios, and confidence intervals

BACKGROUND

If you are working in a group, you will quickly find that some people have a head for figures and others do not. If you are working alone, we suspect you will find this Unit either the easiest in the book or the most difficult. If you are one of the large number of people who find mathematical estimates difficult to conceptualise or calculate, we suggest that you work through this Unit gradually and return to it frequently. You will find that the concepts (which are crucially important) become easier with repetition! Do not allow yourself to be "psyched out" by the ease with which your more numerate colleagues appear to grasp them.

SUGGESTED AIM FOR THIS SESSION

For participants to develop, and feel confident in helping others to develop, a working understanding of the statistical tools for estimating the magnitude and precision of the benefits and harms of therapies.

SUGGESTED LEARNING OBJECTIVES FOR THIS SESSION

By the end of this session, participants should be able to:
- for interventions that produce dichotomous (yes/no) outcomes, calculate the number needed to treat (NNT) for effective therapies and the number needed to harm (NNH) for adverse events and explain the meaning of these terms to others;
- distinguish between relative risk, risk ratio, and odds ratio and explain the meaning of these terms to others;
- determine the confidence interval around the above estimates and explain its significance to others.

SET ARTICLES

1. Sackett DL. On some clinically useful measures of the effects of treatment. *Evidence Based Med* 1996; **1:** 37–8.
2. Sackett DL, Deeks JJ, Altman DG. Down with odds ratios! *Evidence Based Med* 1996; **1:** 164–6.

WORKED EXAMPLE: THE FIRST EVER RANDOMISED CONTROLLED TRIAL (SEE REFERENCE LIST FOR DETAILS)

Background: a rationing decision

Streptomycin, a promising new therapy for tuberculosis, was discovered in 1944 in the USA. The British pound had been devalued so much during the Second World War that anything in dollars was prohibitively expensive. Sir Austin Bradford Hill, working with the Medical Research Council in the UK, secured enough streptomycin to treat only 50 patients. He believed that the only ethical way of distributing this limited quantity of the drug was in a carefully controlled trial in which allocation to experimental and control groups was ensured by random codes in sealed, sequentially numbered envelopes.

Clinical question

What is the efficacy of streptomycin in acute bilateral pulmonary tuberculosis compared with conventional therapy (bed rest)?

Study design

Randomised controlled trial.

Intervention

One hundred consecutive adults presenting with acute bilateral pulmonary tuberculosis were randomly allocated either to streptomycin plus bed rest or bed rest alone.

Main outcome measures

Mortality within the six-month follow-up period; severe adverse drug reactions.

Results

Of 107 adults seen, 52 were allocated to bed rest alone ("control group") and 55 to streptomycin plus bed rest ("experimental group"). The number of deaths was 14 in the control group and four in the experimental group. These figures can be expressed in standard convention as a 2×2 matrix as follows.

	Death from tuberculosis Yes	Death from tuberculosis No	Total
Experimental (streptomycin) group	4 (a)	(b) 51	55
Control group (bed rest alone)	14 (c)	(d) 38	52

The main side effect of the drug was VIIIth nerve damage, leading to permanent deafness. This developed in 36 of the experimental group and none of the control group.

Practical exercise

Using the formulae below, calculate the following.
1. The event rate for death in the control group (CER).

2. The event rate for death in the experimental group (EER).
3. The absolute risk reduction (ARR) with streptomycin therapy.
4. The relative risk reduction (RRR) with streptomycin therapy.
5. The number needed to treat (NNT) for prevention of death with streptomycin therapy.
6. The *risk* (chance) of death in the experimental and control groups respectively.
7. The *odds* of death in the experimental and control groups respectively.
8. The *risk ratio* (relative risk) of death in the experimental group compared with the control group.
9. The *odds ratio* (relative odds) of death in the experimental group compared with the control group.
10. The number needed to harm (NNH) for VIIIth nerve damage on streptomycin.

Note the difference between probability and odds

The probability of something happening is the number of times we believe it is *likely* to occur divided by the number of times we believe it could *possibly* occur.

The odds of something happening is the number of times we believe it is likely to occur divided by the number of times we believe it is likely *not* to occur.

If a couple are expecting a baby, the *probability* of it being a boy is (approximately!) one in two, i.e. 50% or 0.5. The *odds* of the baby being a boy are 1:1 or 1.0, i.e. it is as likely to be a boy as it is not to be a boy.

Formula

	Outcome event		Total
	Yes	No	
Experimental group	a	b	a + b
Control group	c	d	c + d

Control event rate = outcome event rate in control group = CER = c/(c+d)
Experimental event rate = outcome event rate in experimental group = EER = a/(a+b)
Relative risk reduction (RRR) = (CER – EER)/CER
Absolute risk reduction (ARR) = CER – EER
Number needed to treat (NNT) = 1/ARR = 1/(CER – EER)
Relative risk (risk ratio) for death = (a/a+b)/(c/c+d)
Relative odds (odds ratio) for death = (a/b)/(c/d) = ad / bc

For solution see page 160.

A NOTE ON CONFIDENCE INTERVALS

A difference of 20% in the absolute risk of the main outcome variable, corresponding to a number needed to treat of 5 (see page 160), is fairly impressive. But surely this difference might have occurred by chance? Indeed, much larger absolute differences might conceivably occur by chance. Given an infinite amount of funding, time and dedication, these authors could have repeated the same study an infinite number of times and the average result of all the separate trials determined to reflect the "true" difference between the treatment regimens. Since people rarely repeat exactly the same study, the true difference is almost never established empirically. Instead, we call the actual result of one trial the *point estimate of effect size* and calculate the limits within which the "true" result is likely to lie. This latter estimate is known as the *confidence interval*.

The 90%, 95%, and 99% confidence intervals correspond to the limits that have a 90%, 95% or 99% chance respectively of containing the "true" result. Clearly, the 90% confidence interval for any result will be narrower than the 99% interval and although it is perfectly possible to calculate a confidence interval of any percentage you choose, convention prefers the 95% (or, occasionally, 99%) interval.

It makes intuitive sense that the larger the sample size, the narrower the confidence interval (i.e. the more sure you can be that the actual result is pretty close to the "true" difference between the groups). It also makes intuitive sense that an outcome that varies widely in the population will produce a wider confidence interval than one that varies less widely. Hence it should come as no surprise that the three things a statistician needs to know in order to calculate a confidence interval for a particular result are the sample size, the mean and standard deviation of the variable in the population, and the difference obtained in the trial. If the outcome is an event, the percentage in the two groups will be required rather than the mean and the standard deviation.

Most statisticians calculate confidence intervals using a preprogrammed formula on a computer or calculator but if you are curious and wish to produce one from first principles, the formula for a 95% confidence interval is as follows.

Difference in mean value ± 1.96 × standard error of difference in means, or

Difference in percentages ± 1.96 × standard error of difference in percentages.

The number 1.96 is required to make this into a *95%* confidence interval; it would need to be replaced by 2.58 for a 99% confidence interval.

Standard error of difference in means is calculated by the formula:

$$\sqrt{\sigma^2 \times [1/n_1 + 1/n_2]}$$

where n_1 and n_2 are the sample sizes in the two groups.

But σ^2 has to be estimated from the standard deviations in each group. σ^2 is estimated as:

$$\{(n_1 - 1) \times SD_1^2 + (n_2 - 1) \times SD_2^2\} / (n_1 + n_2 - 2)$$

Perhaps you can now see why statisticians prefer a preprogrammed calculator!

FURTHER READING

Bland M. *An introduction to medical statistics.* Oxford: Oxford Medical Publications, 1987.

Bradford Hill A. Streptomycin in pulmonary tuberculosis. *BMJ* 1948: **ii**: 790–1. Available on the Internet on http://www.bmj.com/cgi/content/full/317/7167/1248.

Greenhalgh T. *How to read a paper: the basics of evidence-based medicine.* London: BMJ Books, 1997. See in particular Chapter 5: Statistics for the non-statistician, pages 69–86.

Sackett DL, Cook RJ. The number needed to treat: a clinically useful measure of treatment effect. *BMJ* 1995; **310**: 452–4.

Smeeth L, Haines A, Ebrahim S. Numbers needed to treat derived from meta-analyses – sometimes informative, usually misleading. *BMJ* 1999; **318**: 1548–50.

Evidence Based Medicine

EBM NOTEBOOK
On some clinically useful measures of the effects of treatment

In the abstracts in this journal that describe effective treatments, we provide our readers with numbers that summarise their clinical effect. These include the number of patients you need to treat to prevent 1 adverse outcome (NNT) and both the absolute risk reduction (ARR) and relative risk reduction (RRR) in the occurrence of adverse outcomes achieved by active therapy. In this EBM Note, we explain these numbers for our readers and use them to begin a glossary of terms that will appear in each issue.

In the first issue of *Evidence-Based Medicine*, we presented the results of the Diabetes Control and Complications Trial (DCCT) (1) into the effect of intensive diabetes therapy on the development and progression of neuropathy. In that trial, confirmed neuropathy developed among 9.6% of patients randomly assigned to usual care (1 or 2 insulin injections/d to prevent gylcaemic symptoms; we will call this rate "C" for "control") and among 2.8% of patients randomly assigned to intensive therapy (insulin pump or $\geq$ 3 injections/d; we call this rate "E" for experimental). This difference was statistically highly significant, but how might this treatment effect be expressed in terms of its clinical significance? The traditional measure of this effect is the proportional or "relative" risk reduction (abbreviated RRR in our journal), calculated as (C — E)/C. In this example, the RRR is (9.6%–2.8%)/9.6% or 71%; intensive therapy reduced the risk for developing neuropathy by 71%.

Why not confine our description of the clinical significance of this result to the RRR? The reason is that the RRR fails to discriminate huge absolute treatment effects (10 times those observed in this trial) from those that are trivial (1/10 000 of those observed here). For example, if the rates of neuropathy were 10 times those observed in this trial, and a whopping 96% of control patients and 28% of intensively treated patients developed neuropathy, the RRR would remain unchanged: RRR = (96%–28%)/96% or 71%. And if a trivial 0.00096% of control and 0.00028% of intensively treated patients developed neuropathy, the relative risk reduction is as before: RRR still = (0.00096%–0.00028%)/0.00096 = 71%! This is because the RRR discards the underlying susceptibility (or "baseline risk") of patients entering randomised trials; as a result, the RRR cannot discriminate huge risks and benefits from small ones.

In contrast to these nondiscriminating RRRs, the absolute differences in the rates of neuropathy between control and experimental patients (C — E) clearly do discriminate between these extremes, and this measure is called the absolute risk reduction or ARR. In the DCCT, the ARR or (C — E) = 9.6%–2.8% = 6.8%; in the extremely high hypothetical example, in which 96% of control patients and 28% of intensively treated patients developed neuropathy, the ARR or (C — E) = 96% – 28% = 68%; in the extremely low hypothetical example, in which a trivial 0.00096% of control and 0.00028% of intensively treated patients developed neuropathy, the ARR or (C — E) = 0.00096% – 0.00028% = 0.00068%. These ARRs retain the underlying susceptibility of patients and provide more detailed information than RRRs. But, unlike RRRs that can be recalled as whole numbers, ARRs are decimals and are therefore difficult to remember and do not slip easily off the tongue at the bedside.

If, however, we divide the ARR into 1 (i.e., if we "invert" the ARR or "take its reciprocal" so that it becomes 1/ARR), we generate a very useful number because it represents the number of patients we need to treat (NNT) with the experimental therapy in order to prevent 1 bad outcome. In the DCCT, we would generate the number of persons with diabetes we would need to treat with the intensive regimen in order to prevent 1 from developing neuropathy. In the trial, the NNT is 1/ARR or 1/6.8% or 14.7; we usually round that number upward (in this case, to 15), and we now can say that for every 15 patients who are treated with the more intensive insulin regimen, 1 is prevented from developing diabetic neuropathy.

Is 15 a large or a small number of patients that need to be treated to prevent 1 bad outcome? As with many important matters in medicine, the answer has to do with clinical significance, not statistical significance. This NNT of 15 certainly is far smaller than the number of patients we would need to treat in the extremely low hypothetical example, in which 1/ARR becomes 1/0.00068%, or an NNT of more than 147 000, a figure so vast that we cannot imagine anyone judging it to be worth the effort. We can get a better idea by comparing this NNT of 15 with that for other interventions we are familiar with in medicine. In doing so, we add the dimension of the duration of therapy: in the DCCT, treatment continued for an average of 6.5 years, meaning that we need to treat about 15 persons with diabetes for about 6.5 years with an intensive insulin regimen to prevent 1 from developing neuropathy. How does this compare with other treatments, over other durations, for other conditions?

Beginning on an optimistic note, only about 20 patients with chest pain who appear to be having heart attacks need to be treated with streptokinase and aspirin to save a life at 5 weeks. On the other hand, about 70 elderly persons with hypertension need to

Originally published in *Evidence Based Medicine* 1996; **1**: 37–8.

be treated for 5 years with antihypertensive drugs to save 1 life, about 100 men with no evidence of coronary heart disease need to be treated for 5 years with aspirin to prevent 1 heart attack, and about 10 patients with symptomatic moderate-to-severe carotid artery stenosis need to have endarterectomy to prevent 1 major or fatal stroke over the next 2 years.

We think that the NNT to prevent 1 event is a very useful measure of the clinical effort we and our patients must expend to help them avoid bad outcomes of their illnesses. Accordingly, we will report NNTs in the "Main Results" sections of our abstracts whenever possible. NNTs will be accompanied by the actual event rates and their resultant *P* value and will be followed by their associated RRR.

Furthermore, because we are focusing here on the magnitude of the treatment effect rather than on the probability that we have drawn a false-positive conclusion that the treatment is at all effective (when it is not), we shall report confidence intervals (CIs) around the NNT, specifying the "limits" within which we can confidently state the true NNT lies (95% of the time). Readers who want to brush up on CIs can refer to an earlier editorial

in our companion publication, *ACP Journal Club* (2), and we will also discuss them here in a future EBM Notebook.

Another useful feature of the NNT is the ease with which readers can convert it to NNTs for specific patients in their own practice by using some very simple arithmetic. All the reader needs to do is to estimate the susceptibility (sometimes called the "baseline risk") of her own untreated patient relative to the average control patient in the trial report, and then express this estimate as a decimal fraction we will call "F" (if a reader judged her patient to be twice as susceptible as the average control patient in the trial, then F = 2; if her patient was only half as susceptible, then F = 0.5; and if the patient is as susceptible as the control patients in the trial, then F = 1) (3). If the treatment produces a constant RRR across the spectrum of susceptibilities, the NNT for her patient is simply the reported NNT divided by F. Going back to our intensive insulin example, if a reader's patient was judged to have only half the susceptibility of patients in that trial, then F = 0.5 and NNT/F = 15/0.5 = 30; thus, 30 of these less susceptible patients would need to be

treated for about 6.5 years with the intensive insulin regimen to prevent 1 from developing neuropathy.

This science of the art of extrapolating the results of published reports to individual patients is still in its infancy. We are just beginning to learn how to distinguish situations in which we can (usually with drug treatments) and cannot (sometimes with surgical treatments) assume constant RRRs over the ranges of susceptibilities we commonly encounter, and how to integrate this information with the rest of our clinical findings and clinical judgement. When this learning leads to important advances in our ability to extrapolate from trials to individual patients, we will report them here.

David L. Sackett in Oxford

References
1. Intensive glycaemic control prevented or delayed diabetic neuropathy [Abstract]. EBM. 1995 Nov-Dec;1:9. Abstract of: The Diabetes Control and Complications Trial Group. The effect of intensive diabetes therapy on the development and progression of neuropathy. Ann Intern Med. 1995; 122:561–8.
2. **Altman DG.** Confidence intervals in research evaluation [Editorial]. 1992 Mar-Apr: A28 (Ann Intern Med. vol 116, suppl 2).
3. **Cook RJ, Sackett DL.** The number needed to treat: a clinically useful measure of treatment effect. BMJ. 1995;310:452–4.

Evidence Based Medicine

EBM NOTEBOOK

Down with odds ratios!

As described in an earlier EBM note (1) and in our glossary, this journal reports the results of individual randomised trials in terms of relative risk reductions (RRRs), calculated by dividing the absolute difference in event rates between the control (control event rate [CER]) and experimental (experimental event rate [EER]) patients by the event rate for the controls: (CER − EER)/CER = RRR. From these same values, we also report the number of patients that would need to be treated (NNT) to prevent 1 additional event — 1/(CER − EER) — or by its alternative calculation — 1/(RRR × CER). Thus, in the example shown in Table 1, the RRR is 89% and the NNT is 4(2).

However, we also report the results of overviews of several randomised trials, and these results appear not as RRRs but as relative odds, or odds ratios (ORs). There are reasons for this variation (although, as it happens, arguably no longer very good ones!). We will explain ORs, point out their properties (many of which interfere with their clinical application), and pro-vide you with some practical help in applying them to individual patients.

When used to summarise an overview, an OR describes the odds of an experimental patient having an adverse event relative to a control patient. We can calculate the odds of a patient having an event by dividing the number of patients who have the event by the number of patients who do not. Hence, for the control group in Table 1, the odds of a patient having the event were c/d = 9/21 = 0.43, which compares to a risk of c/(c + d) = 9/30 = 0.30. If we mistakenly interpret odds as if they were risks, we will exaggerate the latter, especially with events that are more common.

The OR is calculated by dividing the odds in the experimental group by the odds in the control group — (a/b)/(c/d) — or equivalently through the "cross-products" calculation shown below Table 1 — ad/bc. From this definition, it follows that efficacious treatments generate ORs < 1, which is analogous to the relative risk (RR) for the adverse event (EER/CER) being < 1. (We usually prefer to think in terms of RRRs, which are equivalent to 1 — RR, but for ease of comparison with ORs, please bear with us and think in terms of RRs.)

How did we get into this confusing situation of using ORs in the first place? The OR had its origins in case-control studies of drug side effects and of harmful agents and exposures, such as cigarette smoking. In these case-control studies, it is not possible to estimate RRs directly because the prevalence of the adverse outcome (required for calculating the RR) is not usually known. You can, however, calculate the OR in these situations, either by comparing the odds of incurring an adverse event in the exposed group and the control group (i.e., [a/b]/[c/d] = ad/bc); or by comparing the odds of exposure in the event and nonevent groups (i.e., [a/c]/[b/d] = ad/bc); both routes lead to the same answer, which will be > 1 when the exposure is harmful. Hence, the OR can be estimated when the prevalence of the events is unknown, as in most case-control studies. Moreover, because case-control studies typically are used for the study of rare events, the distortion of risk produced by interpreting ORs as if they were RRs is negligible (if necessary, refresh your memory by rereading the 3rd paragraph in this note).

When ORs came into use, several powerful and informative statistical methods were developed (by persons such as Nathan Mantel and William Haenszel) for use in analysing subgroups of patients and combining them (even when the latter were unbalanced for confounding factors) into a single overall estimate (3). Later, when scientists began to do overviews of multiple randomised trials and were seeking a statistical method for combining their results, the analogy with combining subgroups in case-control studies was recognised,

Table 1. Trimethoprim-sulfamethoxazole prophylaxis in cirrhosis*

Treatment group	Adverse event (infectious complications)		Totals	
	Occurs	Does not occur		
Experimental (prophylaxis)	1 a	29 b	a+b	30
Control (no prophylaxis)	c 9	d 21	c+d	30
Totals	10 a+c	b+d 50	a+b+c+d	60

*From reference 2.
Control event rate = CER = c/(c+d) = 0.30; experimental event rate = EER = a/(a+b) = 0.033
Control event odds = c/d = 0.43; experimental event odds = a/b = 0.034
Relative risk reduction = RRR = (CER − EER)/CER = 89%
Number needed to treat = NNT = 1/(CER − EER) = 4, also = 1/(RRR × CER) = 4
Relative risk = EER/CER 0.11, also = 1 − RRR = 0.11
Relative odds = odds ratio = OR = (a/b)/(c/d) = ad/bc = 0.08

Originally published in *Evidence Based Medicine* 1996; **1**: 164–6.

and the Mantel-Haenszel method was adapted to this new use (soon joined by a computationally simpler method developed by Richard Peto [4] that provides good approximations to the OR when treatment effects are small and the trials being combined are large and balanced [5]). For these reasons, ORs are now commonly used in the analysis and reporting of overviews of randomised trials that have binary outcomes.

ORs, however, have 5 properties at interfere with their clinical application. First, because very few clinicians are facile at dealing with odds and relative odds, ORs are not useful in their original form at the bedside or in the examining room. Second, in many trials, ORs are not even similar to RRs: In many fields, controlled trials tend to study common adverse events, and it is in these situations that the approximation of the OR to

the RR breaks down. Treating an OR as if it were an accurate estimate of the RR will overestimate both the likely benefits and harms of treatment (6), and this distortion becomes greater as the disease being treated becomes more severe and CERs increase.

Third, and as a result of the foregoing, ORs cannot be used in the same simple way as RRs to calculate the corresponding NNTs for the treatments of interest. To extrapolate results from trials that have different patient expected event rates (PEERs), clinicians need to do separate and complicated calculations of the NNT for each PEER. Although we expect the NNT to decrease as the PEER rises for a treatment with a fixed relative effect, even this is not true for ORs! Looking down a column in Table 2 will show you that, for a fixed OR, the NNT initially decreases as

the PEER rises (as expected), but it increases again when the PEER is above 0.5. This counterintuitive result occurs because the difference between the RR and the OR accelerates as event rates rise.

Fourth, when treatments generate a constant RRR for different CERs (e.g., antihypertensive drugs generate the same RRR for stroke among patients with both severe and mild hypertension), their ORs cannot be constant across these CERs (and vice versa). Finally, when clinicians draw up "league tables" of therapeutic efficacy, the order of treatments based on their RRRs may be different from the order based on ORs when the diseases and disorders in the table are of different severity and have different CERs.
Help is on the way (but not quite here yet). Prospects are very good that meta-analyses do not have to be done by using ORs. Statistical meth-

Table 2. Translating odds ratios to numbers needed to treat*

Patient's expected event rate	Odds ratios								
	0.9	0.85	0.8	0.75	0.7	0.65	0.6	0.55	0.5
0.05	209†	139	104	83	69	59	52	46	41‡
0.10	110	73	54	43	36	31	27	24	21
0.20	61	40	30	24	20	17	14	13	11
0.30	46	30	22	18	14	12	10	9	8
0.40	40	26	19	15	12	10	9	8	7
0.50§	38	25	18	14	11	9	8	7	6
0.70	44	28	20	16	13	10	9	7	6
0.90	101¶	64	46	34	27	22	18	15	12‖

* The numbers in the body of the table are the numbers needed to treat (NNTs) for the corresponding odds ratios (ORs) at that particular patient's expected event rate (PEER). To calculate the NNT for any OR and PEER:

$$NNT = \frac{1 - [PEER \times (1 - OR)]}{PEER \times (1 - OR) \times (1 - PEER)}$$

† The relative risk reduction (RRR) is 10%.
‡ The RRR is 49%.
§ For any OR, the NNT is lowest when the PEER = 0.50.
¶ The RRR is 1%.
‖ The RRR is 9%.

ods for combining both relative risks and absolute risk differences across trials are available (7), although some concern exists that they are not appropriate for all circumstances. Validation work is under way to outline the situations where they can be widely adopted for combining randomised trials into systematic reviews.

As soon as these clinically friendlier alternatives are used in reporting the results of overviews, they will appear in *Evidence-Based Medicine*. In the meantime, we will be adding Table 2 to our glossary, which permits our readers to identify NNTs for a range of ORs and PEERs. The intersection of the OR closest to that reported in the overview with the PEER that best represents the reader's patient will identify the corresponding NNT. For readers who want to do the full calculations, the formula appears below Table 2.

David L. Sackett, MD
NHS Centre for Evidence-Based Medicine
Oxford, England, UK
Jonathan J. Deeks, MSc
Douglas G. Altman, BSc
Centre for Statistics in Medicine
Oxford, England, UK

References
1. **Sackett DL.** On some clinically useful measures of the effects of treatment [EBM note]. *Evidence-Based Medicine.* 1996 Jan-Feb; 1:37–8.
2. **Singh N, Gayowski T, Yu VL, Wagener MM.** Trimethoprim-sulfamethoxazole for the prevention of spontaneous bacterial peritonitis in cirrhosis: a randomized trial. Ann Intern Med. 1995;122:595–8.
3. **Rothman KJ.** Modern Epidemiology. Boston:Little, Brown and Co.; 1986:177–236.
4. **Yusuf S, Peto R, Lewis J, Collins R, Sleight P.** Beta blockade during and after myocardial infarction: overview of the randomized trials. Prog Cardiovasc Dis. 1985; 27:335–71.
5. **Greenland S, Salvan A.** Bias in the onestep method for pooling study results. Stat Med. 1990;9:247–52.
6. **Sinclair JC, Bracken MB.** Clinically useful measures of effect in binary analyses of randomized trials. J Clin Epidemiol. 1994; 47:881–90.
7. **Greenland S, Robins JM.** Estimation of a common effect parameter from sparse follow-up data. Biometrics. 1985;41:55–68.

Papers that address prognosis or harm (cohort studies)

BACKGROUND

In a cohort study, one or more defined groups is followed up to see what happens to them. In a simple *prognosis* study (a type of cohort study), there is only one cohort – people in the early stages of a disease (for example, women with CIN I on cervical smear). Prognosis studies are important because the rational evaluation of a therapeutic intervention (such as a drug or operation) needs to be based on a thorough knowledge of the outcome of the untreated condition. In a *comparative* cohort study (such as the one reprinted here), two groups are studied – one of which has been exposed to a possible harmful agent (in this case, the oral contraceptive pill) and one of which has not.

SUGGESTED AIM FOR THIS SESSION

For participants to develop, and feel confident in helping others to develop, the ability to determine whether the conclusions of an article describing the clinical course and likely outcome of a disorder (prognosis) are both valid and applicable in practice.

SUGGESTED LEARNING OBJECTIVES FOR THIS SESSION

By the end of this session, participants should be able to:
- establish whether a paper claiming to describe a "cohort study" actually used a clearly defined and adequately followed-up inception cohort;
- assess the methodological quality of the study using a structured checklist;
- assess the significance of the results in terms of quantified measures of benefit and harm;
- comment critically on the application and implementation of the results.

SET ARTICLE

Beral V, Hermon C, Kay C, Hannaford P, Darby S, Reeves G. Mortality associated with oral contraceptive use: 25-year follow up of cohort of 46 000 women from the Royal College of General Practitioners' oral contraception study. *BMJ* 1999; **318**: 96–100.

Clinical scenario

Ravina Patel, a 19-year-old student, attends a family planning clinic to seek advice on contraception. She has read a magazine article describing a near-fatal pulmonary embolus in a 35-year-old smoker who took a second-generation contraceptive pill. She is anxious about her own risk of major complications but also keen to use a non-barrier method of contraception if possible.

SUGGESTIONS FOR GROUP EXERCISES

When you have read the paper, try one or more of the following.
1. Make sure everyone in your group understands the figures in the paper and how they were arrived at.
2. Role play a situation in which the family planning nurse explains the prognosis to Ravina and helps her draw up a decision tree depicting the different treatment options.
3. In a simulated teaching scenario, issue this paper to a group of medical or nursing students who have been told "this stuff will be coming up in your end-of-term exams".

SUGGESTION FOR INDIVIDUAL STUDY

Contraception decisions affect almost everyone at some stage in their lives and patients often phrase their questions on this topic in terms such as, "What would *you* do, doctor (nurse)?". Imagine that Ravina was your sister, partner, daughter (or even yourself!). Before you appraise the paper, make a list of the concerns she is likely to raise about the benefits and

---

CRITICAL APPRAISAL CHECKLIST FOR AN ARTICLE DESCRIBING A COHORT STUDY

Note that the questions on the checklist are really looking for problems of bias, confounding, low power, and poor validity.

A. Are the results of the trial valid and do they contain minimum bias?	Yes/No/Don't know
1. Did the trial address a clearly focused question (PEO)? • Population • Exposure to risk factor(s) over specified time period • Outcome(s)	
2. Was the cohort study prospective (stronger) as opposed to retrospective (weaker)?	
3. Were the two groups (control and exposed) similar in relevant factors at the start of the study (e.g. sex, age, social class, smoking)?	
4. Were all the participants who entered the study properly accounted for? • Was follow-up > 80%? If not, is it likely to have affected the results? • Were participants analysed in the groups to which they were initially allocated?	
B. What are the results?	
5. How large was the effect of the exposure? • What outcomes were measured (measures of risk, e.g. odds ratios, relative risk, absolute risk, absolute risk reduction or increase)?	
6. How precise was the estimate of the exposure effect? • What are its confidence limits (or p-values)?	
C. How relevant are the results?	
7. Were the study participants sufficiently different from my population that this study doesn't help me at all?	

harms of oral contraceptives. Now, work through the critical appraisal checklist and then return to this list of concerns. To what extent has your appraisal of the paper enabled you to address them? What additional research studies would you like to have to hand?

FURTHER READING

Donald A, Greenhalgh T. *A hands-on guide to evidence-based health care: practice and implementation*. Oxford: Blackwell Science, 1999.

Greenhalgh T. *How to read a paper: the basics of evidence based medicine*. London: BMJ Books, 1997. See in particular Chapter 3: Getting your bearings, pages 34–52 and Chapter 4: Assessing methodological quality, pages 53–68.

Laupacis A, Wells G, Richardson WS, Tugwell P. Users' guides to the medical literature. V. How to use an article about prognosis. *JAMA* 1994; **271**: 234–7.

Mortality associated with oral contraceptive use: 25 year follow up of cohort of 46 000 women from Royal College of General Practitioners' oral contraception study

Valerie Beral, Carol Hermon, Clifford Kay, Philip Hannaford, Sarah Darby, Gillian Reeves

Editorial by Skegg

Imperial Cancer Research Fund, Cancer Epidemiology Unit, Radcliffe Infirmary, Oxford OX2 6HE
Valerie Beral, *professor*
Carol Hermon, *scientific officer*
Sarah Darby, *professor*
Gillian Reeves, *statistician*

Royal College of General Practitioners, Manchester Research Unit, Parkway House, Manchester M22 4DB
Clifford Kay, *director*
Philip Hannaford, *professor*

Correspondence to: Professor Beral
beral@icrf.icnet.uk

BMJ 1999;318:96–100

Abstract

Objective To describe the long term effects of the use of oral contraceptives on mortality.

Design Cohort study with 25 year follow up. Details of oral contraceptive use and of morbidity and mortality were reported six monthly by general practitioners. 75% of the original cohort was "flagged" on the NHS central registers.

Setting 1400 general practices throughout Britain.

Subjects 46 000 women, half of whom were using oral contraceptives at recruitment in 1968-9. Median age at end of follow up was 49 years.

Main outcome measures Relative risks of death adjusted for age, parity, social class, and smoking.

Results Over the 25 year follow up 1599 deaths were reported. Over the entire period of follow up the risk of death from all causes was similar in ever users and never users of oral contraceptives (relative risk = 1.0, 95% confidence interval 0.9 to 1.1; P = 0.7) and the risk of death for most specific causes did not differ significantly in the two groups. However, among current and recent (within 10 years) users the relative risk of death from ovarian cancer was 0.2 (0.1 to 0.8; P = 0.01), from cervical cancer 2.5 (1.1 to 6.1; P = 0.04), and from cerebrovascular disease 1.9 (1.2 to 3.1, P = 0.009). By contrast, for women who had stopped use ≥ 10 years previously there were no significant excesses or deficits either overall or for any specific cause of death.

Conclusion Oral contraceptives seem to have their main effect on mortality while they are being used and in the 10 years after use ceases. Ten or more years after use ceases mortality in past users is similar to that in never users.

Introduction

Oral contraceptives have been available for 40 years and, although their short term effects on health have been studied in detail,[1][2] comparatively little is known about whether these effects persist after use stops. The Royal College of General Practitioners' oral contraception study was set up in 1968 to monitor the health of women who had used oral contraceptives. We present the results of a 25 year follow up of that population examining the effect of use of oral contraceptives on mortality in the long term.

Subjects and methods

Over 14 months from May 1968, 1400 general practitioners throughout the United Kingdom recruited 23 000 women who were using oral contraceptives and a similar number who had never used them into the oral contraception study.[1] Most women (98%) were white and all were married or living as married. General practitioners were asked to provide information on oral contraceptives prescribed, pregnancies, new illness, or death for each subject every six months. During the early years of the study some general practitioners withdrew their patients and some women moved and left the study. In 1976-7 an attempt was made to "flag" the cohort on the NHS central registers in Southport and Edinburgh to provide information on death and cause of death for women who were no longer being followed regularly by their general practitioner. About 75% of the original cohort was successfully flagged, and these women have been followed for death and emigration since then. The remaining 25% could not be flagged because they or their general practitioners had left the study before the flagging procedure could be instigated and the personal details required for flagging were not available to the investigators. The mortality of the women who were followed regularly by their general practitioner was similar to that of women who left the study.[3]

This analysis includes deaths up to 31 December 1993. We obtained a copy of the death certificate for all women who had died, and CK or PH coded the cause of death according to ICD-8 (international classification of diseases, eighth revision),[4] occasionally supplementing information from the death certificate with details provided by general practitioners.[5] Person-years of follow up were calculated from the date of recruitment up to the date of death for the 1599 women who had died, up to the date of last contact with the general practitioner for 10 958 women who were not flagged on the NHS registers, or up to 31 December 1993 for 33 554 women who were flagged on the NHS registers and alive on that date.[3] For women who were no longer being followed by their general practitioner before 1 January 1977 but were

Originally published in *BMJ* 1999; **318**: 96–100.

flagged no person-years were included for the period between the date of last contact with their general practitioner and 1 January 1977 because the ascertainment of deaths during that period may have been incomplete.[3]

Person-years were categorised by age (16-19, 20-24...70-79), parity (0, 1-2, ≥3, not known), social class at recruitment (I-II, III, IV-V, other), and cigarette smoking at recruitment (0, 1-14/day, ≥15/day, not known) with a standard computer program.[6] Person-years were further subdivided according to whether the women had taken oral contraceptives and, where appropriate, by duration of use and time since first and last use. At recruitment half (23 000) of the subjects were using oral contraceptives, but by 31 December 1993, 63% had used them at some time. Women who started using oral contraceptives after recruitment contributed person-years to the "never user" category up to the date that they began using them. For women who were flagged on the NHS registers but no longer regularly followed up by their general practitioner, we assumed that past users and never users who were over the age of 40 at the date of last contact did not subsequently take oral contraceptives. For current users and women aged under 40 at the time of last contact with their general practitioners, we assumed that use continued for two years as stated at the time of last contact, but thereafter use was classified as unknown. These assumptions about subsequent use of oral contraceptives are similar to those used in analyses of other cohort studies.[7]

The results presented here are based on 853 517 person-years of follow up until 31 December 1993: 517 519 in women who had used oral contraceptives and 335 998 in women who had never used them. Standardised mortality ratios were calculated by using mortality for women in England and Wales as a standard.[6] Relative risks were adjusted for age, parity, social class, and smoking with the Poisson regression program module of EPICURE.[8] P values are two tailed.

Results

By 31 December 1993 the cohort had been followed for 25 years and the median age of the women was 49 years (48 for ever users of oral contraception and 50 for never users). During that period 1599 deaths were reported, 945 in ever users and 654 in never users (table 1). The death rate from all causes combined was 21% lower than in the UK population (overall standardised mortality ratio = 79). The relative risk of death from all causes combined after adjustment for age, parity, social class, and cigarette smoking did not differ significantly between ever users and never users (relative risk = 1.0, 95% confidence interval 0.9 to 1.1; P = 0.7).

Table 1 also shows standardised mortality ratios and adjusted relative risks of death for common specific causes and groups of causes of death (and also for some particular causes that have been reported to be affected by oral contraceptive use) according to ever use of oral contraceptives. For most specific causes of death the standardised mortality ratios in ever users and never users of oral contraceptives were around 100 and did not differ significantly between the two groups. The few exceptions were colorectal cancer and

Table 1 Standardised mortality ratios in ever users and never users of oral contraceptives and relative risk in ever users compared with never users

Cause of death (ICD-8 code)	Standardised mortality ratio (No of deaths)		Relative risk† (95% CI)
	Ever users	Never users	
All causes (000-999)	82 (945)	74 (654)	1.0 (0.9 to 1.1)
All cancers (140-209)	85 (474)	85 (355)	1.0 (0.8 to 1.1)
Colorectal (153-154)	62 (29)	108 (39)	0.6 (0.4 to 0.9)*
Liver (155)	126 (5)	34 (1)	5.0 (0.6 to 43.2)
Lung (162)	107 (75)	71 (40)	1.2 (0.8 to 1.8)
Breast (174)	87 (154)	81 (105)	1.1 (0.8 to 1.4)
Cervix (180)	115 (38)	57 (13)	1.7 (0.9 to 3.2)
Uterus (181-2)	22 (2)	83 (6)	0.3 (0.1 to 1.4)
Ovary (183)	49 (24)	83 (31)	0.6 (0.3 to 1.0)*
Other cancers	87 (147)	95 (120)	0.9 (0.7 to 1.1)
All circulatory diseases (390-458)	84 (237)	63 (143)	1.2 (1.0 to 1.5)
Ischaemic heart disease (410-4)	70 (98)	68 (79)	0.9 (0.7 to 1.3)
Other heart disease (420-9)	107 (19)	66 (9)	1.4 (0.6 to 3.1)
Cerebrovascular disease (430-8)	111 (87)	62 (38)	1.5 (1.0 to 2.3)*
Other circulatory	73 (33)	46 (17)	1.4 (0.8 to 2.5)
All digestive diseases (520-77)	85 (37)	74 (24)	1.1 (0.6 to 1.8)
Liver disease (570-3)	112 (23)	69 (10)	1.7 (0.8 to 3.6)
All other diseases (1-139, 210-389, 460-519, 578-799)	53 (95)	65 (89)	0.8 (0.6 to 1.0)
Violent or accidental causes (800-999)	111 (102)	68 (43)	1.6 (1.1 to 2.3)*
Suicide (950-9)	123 (39)	73 (16)	1.5 (0.8 to 2.7)

*P<0.05. †Adjusted for age, social class, parity, and smoking.

ovarian cancer, for which the relative risks of death in users were significantly below 1.0, and cerebrovascular disease and all violent and accidental causes of death, for which the relative risks were significantly greater than 1.0. Ever use is, however, a crude measure of use of oral contraceptives.

Table 2 shows for various causes the relative risk of death compared with never users in relation to the number of years since oral contraceptives were first used. Within the first 10 years of starting use of oral contraceptives there was a significant excess mortality from all causes of death (relative risk = 1.2, 95% confidence interval 1.0 to 1.50; P = 0.03), all circulatory diseases (2.2, 1.5 to 3.2; P < 0.0001), and cerebrovascular disease (2.7, 1.5 to 4.9; P = 0.0008). However, the excess mortality from these causes fell with time, this trend being significant for all circulatory disease (P = 0.002) and cerebrovascular disease (P = 0.02). There were 380 deaths in women who began using oral contraceptives more than 20 years before the end of follow up, and this group showed no significant excess or deficit in mortality from any specific condition or overall.

Table 3 shows the pattern of risk of death for various conditions in relation to the time since stopping use of oral contraceptives. By the end of follow up the median time since last use in the cohort was 17 years. Significant increases or decreases in risk were found mainly in current users or those who had stopped use within the past 10 years—for example, women who were current users or who stopped use in the past five years had a significantly reduced risk of ovarian cancer (0.1, 0.0 to 0.9; P = 0.04) and a significant excess of all circulatory diseases (1.7, 1.2 to 2.4; P = 0.006) and cerebrovascular disease (1.9, 1.1 to 3.4; P = 0.03) and women who had stopped use five to nine years previously had an significant excess risk of cervical cancer (3.0, 1.1 to 8.1; P = 0.03) and cerebrovascular disease (2.0, 1.1 to 3.7; P = 0.02). Among women who had stopped use 15 or more years previously most of

Table 2 Relative risk of death in users of oral contraceptives compared with never users according to time since first use

| Cause of death (ICD-8 code) | Years since first use of oral contraceptives | | | | | | (P value) test for trend by time since first use |
| | <10 | | 10-19 | | ≥20 | | |
	Relative risk† (95% CI)	No of deaths	Relative risk† (95% CI)	No of deaths	Relative risk† (95% CI)	No of deaths	
All causes (000-999)	1.2 (1.0 to 1.5)*	167	1.1 (0.9 to 1.2)	398	0.9 (0.8 to 1.1)	380	0.09
All cancers (140-209)	0.9 (0.7 to 1.3)	61	1.0 (0.8 to 1.2)	212	0.9 (0.8 to 1.1)	201	0.6
Colorectal (153-154)	0.7 (0.2 to 2.2)	4	0.5 (0.3 to 1.1)	11	0.6 (0.3 to 1.1)	14	0.8
Lung (162)	0.9 (0.3 to 2.3)	5	1.3 (0.8 to 2.1)	34	1.2 (0.7 to 1.9)	36	0.8
Breast (174)	1.1 (0.7 to 1.8)	22	1.2 (0.9 to 1.6)	74	1.0 (0.7 to 1.3)	58	0.8
Cervix (180)	0.8 (0.3 to 2.5)	5	2.0 (1.00 to 4.0)	22	1.8 (0.8 to 4.2)	11	0.2
Ovary (183)	0.9 (0.3 to 2.7)	4	0.5 (0.2 to 1.0)*	8	0.6 (0.3 to 1.3)	12	0.8
Other cancers	1.0 (0.6 to 1.6)	21	0.9 (0.7 to 1.2)	63	0.9 (0.7 to 1.2)	70	0.4
All circulatory diseases (390-458)	2.2 (1.5 to 3.2)**	49	1.3 (1.0 to 1.7)	99	0.9 (0.7 to 1.2)	89	0.002
Ischaemic heart disease (410-414)	1.8 (1.0 to 3.2)	14	1.0 (0.7 to 1.6)	41	0.8 (0.5 to 1.1)	43	0.02
Other heart disease (420-429)	2.1 (0.5 to 9.3)	3	1.7 (0.6 to 4.5)	8	1.1 (0.4 to 3.0)	8	0.7
Cerebrovascular disease (430-438)	2.7(1.5 to 4.9)**	23	1.7 (1.1 to 2.7)*	39	1.0 (0.6 to 1.8)	25	0.02
Other circulatory	2.4 (0.9 to 6.5)	9	1.2 (0.6 to 2.7)	11	1.2 (0.6 to 2.5)	13	0.9
All digestive diseases (520-577)	1.2 (0.5 to 3.0)	7	1.3 (0.7 to 2.4)	18	0.9 (0.4 to 1.8)	12	0.9
Liver disease (570-573)	2.0 (0.6 to 7.0)	4	1.5 (0.6 to 3.7)	9	1.8 (0.7 to 4.4)	10	0.7
All other diseases (1-139, 210-389, 460-519, 578-799)	0.9 (0.5 to 1.6)	16	0.6 (0.4 to 0.9)*	28	0.9 (0.6 to 1.3)	51	0.4
Violent and accidental causes (800-999)	1.6 (1.0 to 2.7)	34	1.5 (1.0 to 2.3)	41	1.6 (1.0 to 2.7)	27	0.9
Suicide (950-959)	1.9 (0.9 to 4.1)	16	1.4 (0.7 to 2.8)	17	1.1 (0.4 to 2.9)	6	0.2

*P<0.05,**P<0.01. †Adjusted for age, parity, social class, and smoking.

the relative risks were around 1.0. For ovarian cancer there was a weak suggestion that the protective effect associated with current or recent use wore off (test for trend, P = 0.05).

Among ever users of oral contraceptives, the average duration of use was five years. Table 4 shows the relative risk of death in relation to the duration of use of oral contraceptives. Women who used oral contraceptives for 10 or more years had a significant excess mortality from lung cancer (2.0, 1.1 to 3.5; P = 0.02) and cervical cancer (4.1, 1.6 to 10.6; P = 0.003). The excess deaths from lung cancer were mainly among smokers (17 deaths in smokers and three in non-smokers), the relative risk associated with 10 or more years of use of oral contraceptives being 2.0

for smokers and 2.2 for non-smokers. This excess may be a chance finding or perhaps due to residual confounding. There was also a significant trend of increasing mortality for all cancers combined and for cervical cancer in relation to duration of use (P = 0.02 and 0.03, respectively).

Duration of use and time since first and last use of oral contraceptives were highly correlated, with current and recent users being more likely to have used contraceptives for longer. Table 5 shows the relative risk of death among ever users of oral contraceptives according to time since last use of oral contraceptives and duration of use. All significant results were confined to women currently using oral contraceptives or who had stopped in the past 10 years, although

Table 3 Relative risk of death in users of oral contraceptives compared with never users according to time since last use

| Cause of death (ICD-8 codes) | Years since last use of oral contraceptives | | | | | | | | (P value) test for trend by time since last use |
| | Current and <5 | | 5-9 | | 10-14 | | ≥15 | | |
	Relative risk† (95% CI)	No of deaths	Relative risk† (95% CI)	No of deaths	Relative risk† (95% CI)	No of deaths	Relative risk† (95% CI)	No of deaths	
All causes (000-999)	1.0 (0.9 to 1.2)	199	1.1 (0.9 to 1.3)	142	1.1 (0.9 to 1.3)	189	0.9 (0.8 to 1.1)	196	1.0
All cancers (140-209)	0.9 (0.7 to 1.1)	81	1.1 (0.8 to 1.4)	79	1.1 (0.8 to 1.3)	104	0.9 (0.7 to 1.1)	99	0.9
Colorectal (153-154)	0.5 (0.2 to 1.4)	4	0.6 (0.2 to 1.6)	4	0.2 (0.1 to 0.8)*	2	1.0 (0.5 to 2.0)	12	0.1
Lung (162)	0.8 (0.3 to 1.7)	8	1.1 (0.6 to 2.2)	11	1.3 (0.8 to 2.4)	19	1.2 (0.6 to 2.1)	18	0.9
Breast (174)	1.0 (0.6 to 1.6)	28	1.5 (1.0 to 2.2)	31	1.3 (0.8 to 1.9)	33	0.9 (0.6 to 1.5)	25	0.8
Cervix (180)	2.2 (0.8 to 6.1)	9	3.0 (1.1 to 8.1)*	8	1.6 (0.5 to 4.9)	5	0.7 (0.1 to 3.2)	2	0.3
Ovary (183)	0.1 (0.0 to 0.9)*	1	0.3 (0.1 to 1.4)	2	0.7 (0.3 to 1.8)	6	0.7 (0.3 to 1.7)	6	0.05
Other cancers	1.0 (0.6 to 1.6)	31	0.9 (0.6 to 1.4)	23	1.1 (0.7 to 1.6)	39	0.8 (0.6 to 1.2)	36	0.4
All circulatory diseases (390-458)	1.7 (1.2 to 2.4)**	56	1.4 (0.9 to 2.0)	36	1.2 (0.8 to 1.7)	45	1.0 (0.7 to 1.4)	52	0.2
Ischaemic heart disease (410-414)	1.5 (0.8 to 2.8)	17	0.7 (0.3 to 1.4)	9	1.0 (0.6 to 1.6)	19	1.0 (0.6 to 1.6)	30	0.6
Other heart disease (420-429)	2.4 (0.6 to 9.7)	4	3.0 (0.9 to 10.7)	4	0.7 (0.2 to 3.4)	2	1.0 (0.3 to 3.0)	5	0.3
Cerebrovascular disease (430-438)	1.9 (1.1 to 3.4)*	26	2.0 (1.1 to 3.7)*	18	1.4 (0.8 to 2.6)	16	1.0 (0.5 to 1.9)	13	0.2
Other circulatory	1.8 (0.6 to 4.9)	9	1.7 (0.6 to 4.9)	5	1.8 (0.7 to 4.3)	8	0.1 (0.2 to 2.2)	4	0.6
All digestive diseases (520-577)	1.1 (0.4 to 2.7)	8	1.1 (0.4 to 2.9)	5	1.4 (0.6 to 3.3)	8	0.8 (0.3 to 2.1)	5	0.4
Liver disease (570-573)	1.3 (0.4 to 4.6)	4	2.0 (0.6 to 6.9)	4	1.8 (0.5 to 6.1)	4	1.7 (0.5 to 5.8)	4	0.5
All other diseases (1-139,210-389, 460-519, 578-799)	0.6 (0.3 to 1.1)	19	0.6 (0.3 to 1.1)	10	0.8 (0.5 to 1.3)	19	0.8 (0.5 to 1.3)	28	0.4
Violent and accidental causes (800-999)	1.3 (0.8 to 2.1)	35	1.3 (0.7 to 2.6)	12	1.5 (0.8 to 2.8)	13	1.5 (0.8 to 3.1)	12	0.6
Suicide (950-959)	1.4 (0.6 to 3.0)	16	1.5 (0.6 to 3.9)	6	1.2 (0.4 to 3.7)	4	1.2 (0.3 to 4.5)	3	0.7

*P<0.05, **P<0.01. †Adjusted for age, parity, social class, and smoking.

Table 4 Relative risk of death in users of oral contraceptives compared with never users according to duration of use

Cause of death (ICD-8 code)	Duration of oral contraceptive use (years)						(P value) test for trend with duration of use
	<5		5-9		≥10		
	Relative risk† (95% CI)	No of deaths	Relative risk† (95% CI)	No of deaths	Relative risk† (95% CI)	No of deaths	
All causes (000-999)	1.0 (0.9 to 1.1)	359	1.0 (0.9 to 1.2)	226	1.1 (0.9 to 1.3)	141	0.2
All cancers (140-209)	0.9 (0.7 to 1.1)	167	0.9 (0.7 to 1.1)	108	1.3 (1.0 to 1.6)	88	0.02
Colorectal (153-154)	0.6 (0.3 to 1.2)	11	0.8 (0.4 to 1.6)	9	0.3 (0.1 to 1.2)	2	0.6
Lung (162)	1.1 (0.6 to 1.8)	25	0.7 (0.4 to 1.4)	11	2.0 (1.1 to 3.5)*	20	0.1
Breast (174)	1.1 (0.8 to 1.6)	58	1.0 (0.7 to 1.5)	33	1.4 (0.9 to 2.1)	26	0.4
Cervix (180)	1.3 (0.5 to 3.4)	9	1.4 (0.5 to 4.0)	6	4.1 (1.6 to 10.6)**	9	0.03
Ovary (183)	0.5 (0.2 to 1.2)	8	0.6 (0.3 to 1.5)	6	0.2 (0.0 to 1.3)	1	0.5
Other cancers	0.8 (0.6 to 1.1)	56	1.0 (0.7 to 1.4)	43	1.2 (0.8 to 1.8)	30	0.1
All circulatory diseases (390-458)	1.2 (0.9 to 1.6)	95	1.3 (1.0 to 1.8)	66	1.0 (0.7 to 1.6)	28	0.6
Ischaemic heart disease (410-414)	1.0 (0.7 to 1.6)	38	1.0 (0.7 to 1.7)	25	0.8 (0.5 to 1.6)	12	0.6
Other heart disease (420-429)	1.2 (0.4 to 3.3)	7	2.1 (0.8 to 5.7)	7	0.5 (0.1 to 4.2)	1	1.0
Cerebrovascular disease (430-438)	1.5 (0.9 to 2.3)	35	1.7 (1.0 to 2.9)*	27	1.3 (0.7 to 2.6)	11	0.9
Other circulatory	1.5 (0.7 to 3.2)	15	1.2 (0.5 to 3.0)	7	1.4 (0.4 to 4.2)	4	0.8
All digestive diseases (520-577)	1.1 (0.5 to 2.2)	14	0.9 (0.4 to 2.2)	7	1.2 (0.4 to 3.3)	5	1.0
Liver disease (570-573)	1.4 (0.5 to 3.8)	7	1.4 (0.4 to 4.7)	4	3.0 (1.0 to 9.5)	5	0.3
All other diseases (1-139, 210-389, 460-519, 578-799)	0.8 (0.5 to 1.1)	41	0.8 (0.5 to 1.2)	25	0.5 (0.3 to 1.1)	10	0.6
Violent and accidental causes (800-999)	1.4 (0.9 to 2.1)	42	1.3 (0.8 to 2.3)	20	1.4 (0.7 to 2.9)	10	0.9
Suicide (950-959)	1.1 (0.5 to 2.4)	14	1.8 (0.8 to 3.9)	11	1.4 (0.5 to 4.5)	4	0.4

*P<0.05, **P<0.01. †Adjusted for age, parity, social class, and smoking.

among such women duration of use was not associated with a significant increase or decrease in mortality from any particular cause or overall. Women who stopped using oral contraceptives 10 or more years previously had no significant increases or decreases in relative risk of death from any cause, even if they had used them for 10 years or more. There were, however, only 54 deaths in this subgroup.

Discussion

Our results suggest that most of the effects of oral contraceptives on mortality occur in current or recent users and that few, if any, effects persist 10 years after stopping use. These results relate predominantly to use of combined oral contraceptives containing 50 µg oestrogen.[1]

Information on use of oral contraceptives was recorded prospectively at six monthly intervals by the subjects' general practitioner and so is unlikely to be biased by subsequent events. Furthermore, because three quarters of the original cohort was "flagged" on the NHS central registers in England and Scotland and so followed routinely for death, the findings are likely to be representative of the majority of the women originally recruited. Mortality was similar in women

Table 5 Relative risk† of death in users of oral contraceptives compared with never users according to time since last use and duration of use

Cause of death (ICD-8 code)	Current users or last use <10 years previously			Last use ≥10 years previously		
	All users (95% CI)	Duration of use <10 years (No of deaths)	Duration of use ≥10 years (No of deaths)	All users (95% CI)	Duration of use <10 years (No of deaths)	Duration of use ≥10 years (No of deaths)
All causes (000-999)	1.0 (0.9 to 1.2)	1.0 (254)	1.1 (87)	1.0 (0.9 to 1.1)	1.0 (331)	1.1 (54)
All cancers (140-209)	1.0 (0.8 to 1.2)	0.8 (104)	1.3 (56)	1.0 (0.8 to 1.2)	1.0 (171)	1.2 (32)
Colorectal (153-154)	0.5 (0.2 to 1.2)	0.5 (6)	0.5 (2)	0.6 (0.3 to 1.2)	0.7 (14)	0.0 (0)
Lung (162)	0.9 (0.5 to 1.7)	0.6 (9)	1.6 (10)	1.2 (0.8 to 2.0)	1.1 (27)	2.6 (10)
Breast (174)	1.2 (0.8 to 1.7)	1.1 (40)	1.5 (19)	1.1 (0.8 to 1.5)	1.1 (51)	1.1 (7)
Cervix (180)	2.5 (1.1 to 6.1)*	1.6 (9)	5.3 (8)	1.1 (0.4 to 3.1)	1.2 (6)	1.5 (1)
Ovary (183)	0.2 (0.1 to 0.7)*	0.2 (2)	0.3 (1)	0.7 (0.4 to 1.4)	0.8 (12)	0.0 (0)
Other cancers	0.9 (0.7 to 1.3)	0.9 (38)	1.1 (16)	0.9 (0.7 to 1.3)	0.9 (61)	1.3 (14)
All circulatory diseases(390-458)	1.5 (1.1 to 2.0)**	1.7 (76)	1.1 (16)	1.1 (0.8 to 1.4)	1.1 (85)	1.0 (12)
Ischaemic heart disease (410-414)	1.0 (0.6 to 1.7)	1.2 (21)	0.7 (5)	1.0 (0.7 to 1.5)	1.0 (42)	1.1 (7)
Other heart disease (420-429)	2.8 (0.9 to 8.4)	3.5 (7)	1.3 (1)	0.9 (0.3 to 2.4)	1.0 (7)	0.0 (0)
Cerebrovascular disease (430-438)	1.9 (1.2 to 3.1)*	2.1 (36)	1.5 (8)	1.2 (0.7 to 2.0)	1.2 (26)	1.0 (3)
Other circulatory	1.7 (0.7 to 3.9)	1.8 (12)	1.2 (2)	1.2 (0.5 to 2.7)	1.1 (10)	1.5 (2)
All digestive diseases (520-577)	1.0 (0.5 to 2.2)	0.9 (9)	1.5 (4)	1.1 (0.5 to 2.2)	1.1 (12)	0.7 (1)
Liver disease (570-573)	1.6 (0.6 to 4.4)	1.0 (4)	3.6 (4)	1.7 (0.6 to 4.7)	1.8 (7)	1.9 (1)
All other diseases (1-139, 210-389, 460-519, 578-799)	0.6 (0.4 to 1.0)*	0.7 (25)	0.4 (4)	0.8 (0.6 to 1.2)	0.8 (41)	0.8 (6)
Violent and accidental causes (800-999)	1.3 (0.8 to 2.0)	1.3 (40)	1.4 (7)	1.5 (0.9 to 2.6)	1.5 (22)	1.8 (3)
Suicide (950-959)	1.4 (0.7 to 2.9)	1.4 (19)	1.3 (3)	1.2 (0.5 to 3.1)	1.1 (6)	1.9 (1)

*P<0.05,**P<0.01. †Adjusted for age, parity, social class, and smoking. No significant differences in relative risk were found between women who used oral contraceptives for <10 and ≥10 years.

who remained under regular follow up by their general practitioner and in women who did not.[3] That overall mortality in our cohort was about 20% below the national average is not unexpected since women with severe chronic illnesses were not recruited.[1 3]

Death certificates were obtained for all women who died. There was good agreement between cause of death recorded on the death certificate and that reported by general practitioners.[5] We adjusted for the potential confounding factors of age, parity, social class, and cigarette smoking. Information on age and parity was updated throughout the follow up, whereas social class and smoking details were recorded at entry only. Information on subsequent smoking habits was obtained in 1994-5 for 11 797 members of the original cohort; re-estimation of the risk of myocardial infarction associated with oral contraceptive use based on the updated data gave virtually identical results to those based on smoking history at entry.[9] Use of information on smoking at entry is thus unlikely to have biased our results. We did not adjust for hypertension or other heart disease because such conditions could be in the causal pathway for death from circulatory diseases. No data on family history of these conditions or of cancer were available, but the absence of such information is unlikely to produce spurious associations suggesting that mortality varies according to the timing of oral contraceptive use.

The specific diseases showing significant excesses or deficits in mortality in our study were generally consistent with the results of other studies on the incidence of these diseases.[1 2 10] Other cohort studies have reported no significant changes in mortality among women who have ever used oral contraceptives, which might at first sight be interpreted as inconsistent with their known effects on incidence of disease.[11 12] What our results highlight, however, is that the effects of oral contraceptives on mortality occur mainly in current and recent users.

The effects of oral contraceptives on circulatory diseases are already recognised to be largely confined to current users, especially if they also smoke.[13-16] There has been concern, however, that oral contraceptive use might affect risk of cancer many years after use stops. The collaborative reanalysis of the worldwide data on the relation between breast cancer and oral contraceptive use, which included data from this study, showed that the incidence of breast cancer was slightly increased while women used oral contraceptives and in the 10 years after stopping use but that there was no excess risk 10 or more years after stopping.[7] Our results are consistent with this finding and suggest that other cancers of the female reproductive organs may also be affected by current and recent use of oral contraceptives but may wear off after use stops. The number of deaths from each type of cancer was small, and further data are needed to confirm our findings. Continued follow up of this and other cohorts will yield important information for the many millions of women throughout the world who have used oral contraceptives.

We thank the 1400 doctors who have contributed data to the study.

Contributors: CK set up the oral contraception study and PH took over as director in 1994. CH, SD, GR, and VB contributed to the data analysis. VB prepared the first draft of the manuscript and all other authors have contributed to it. CK is guarantor for the quality of the data; VB and CH are guarantors for the analyses and text.

Funding: Royal College of General Practitioners, British Heart Foundation, Imperial Cancer Research Fund, Medical Insurance Agency, Medical Research Council, Schering AG (Berlin), Schering Health Care (UK), Searle, and Wyeth-Ayerst International (USA).

Competing interests: None declared.

<table>
<tr><td>Key messages</td></tr>
</table>

Key messages

- This 25 year follow up of 46 000 UK women found a decrease in mortality from ovarian cancer and an increase in mortality from circulatory diseases and cervical cancer among women were using oral contraceptives or had used them in the past 10 years

- 10 or more years after stopping use mortality was similar in past users and never users

- Oral contraceptives seem to have their main effect on mortality mainly while they are being used and in the 10 years after stopping use

- There is little evidence to suggest any persistent adverse effect 10 or more years after use of oral contraceptives ceases

1   Royal College of General Practitioners. *Oral contraceptives and health.* London: Pitman Medical, 1974.
2   Vessey M, Doll R, Peto R, Johnson B, Wiggins P. A long-term follow-up study of women using different methods of contraception—an interim report. *J Biosoc Sci* 1976;8:373-427.
3   Beral V, Hermon C, Kay C, Hannaford P, Darby S, Reeves G. Mortality in relation to method of follow up in the Royal College of General Practitioners' oral contraception study. In: Hannaford PS, Webb AMC, eds. *Evidence-guided prescribing of the pill.* London: Parthenon Publishing, 1996:327-39.
4   World Health Organisation. *International classification of diseases, injuries and causes of death: 8th revision, 1965.* Geneva: WHO, 1967.
5   Wingrave SJ, Beral V, Adelstein AM, Kay CR. Comparison of cause of death coding on death certificates with coding in the Royal College of General Practitioners' oral contraception study. *J Epidemiol Community Health* 1981;35:51-8.
6   Coleman M, Douglas A, Hermon C, Peto J. Cohort study analysis with a FORTRAN computer program. *Int J Epidemiol* 1986;15:134-7.
7   Collaborative Group on Hormonal Factors in Breast Cancer. Breast cancer and hormonal contraceptives: collaborative reanalysis of individual data of 53 297 women with breast cancer and 100 239 women without breast cancer from 54 epidemiological studies. *Lancet* 1996;347:1713-27.
8   Preston DL, Lubin JH, Pierce DA. *EPICURE users' guide.* Seattle, WA: Hirosoft International, 1993.
9   Owen-Smith V, Hannaford PC, Warskyj M, Ferry S, Kay CR. Effects of changes in smoking status on risk estimates for myocardial infarction among women recruited for the Royal College of General Practitioners' oral contraception study in the UK. *J Epidemiol Community Health* (in press).
10 Vessey MP. The Jephcott lecture, 1989. An overview of the benefits and risks of combined oral contraceptives. In: Mann RD, ed. *Oral contraceptives and breast cancer.* Park Ridge, NJ: Parthenon Press, 1990:1221-32.
11 Vessey MP, Villard-Mackintosh L, McPherson K, Yeates D. Mortality among oral contraceptive users: 20 year follow up of women in a cohort study. *BMJ* 1989;299:1487-91.
12 Colditz GA. Oral contraceptive use and mortality during 12 years of follow-up: the nurses' health study. *Ann Intern Med* 1994;120:821-6.
13 Royal College of General Practitioners' Oral Contraception Study. Incidence of arterial disease among oral contraceptive users. *J R Coll Gen Pract* 1983;33:75-82.
14 World Health Organisation Collaborative Study of Cardiovascular Disease and Steroid Hormone Contraception. Ischaemic stroke and combined oral contraceptives. Haemorrhagic stroke and overall stroke risk and combined oral contraceptives: results of an international, multicentre, case-control study. *Lancet* 1996;348:498-510.
15 World Health Organisation Collaborative Study of Cardiovascular Disease and Steroid Hormone Contraception. Acute myocardial infarction and combined oral contraceptives: results of an international multicentre case-control study. *Lancet* 1997;349:1202-9.
16 World Health Organisation Scientific Group. Cardiovascular disease and steroid hormone contraception. *WHO Tech Rep Ser* 1998;877.

(Accepted 15 September 1998)

Papers that report diagnostic or screening tests

BACKGROUND

Clinicians increasingly order diagnostic and screening tests and health service users increasingly expect them. But tests are never 100% accurate and the "false-positive" and "false-negative" result carries its own morbidity.

SUGGESTED AIM FOR THIS SESSION

This unit is intended to allow participants to develop, and feel confident in helping others to develop, the ability to evaluate a study to determine the performance of a diagnostic or screening test against an established gold standard and decide on its usefulness in practice.

SUGGESTED LEARNING OBJECTIVES FOR THIS SESSION

By the end of this session, participants should be able to approach a published paper about a diagnostic or screening test with a view to extracting and using the following data.
- What is the *prevalence (pre-test likelihood)* of the disease in this population?
- If a patient really had the disease, what is the likelihood that the test will be positive (*sensitivity*)?
- If a patient really did not have the disease, what is the likelihood that the test will be negative (*specificity*)?
- If the patient tests positive for a particular disease, what is the likelihood that he/she really has the disease (*post-test likelihood of a positive test*)?
- If the patient tests negative for the disease, what is the likelihood that he/she really does not have the disease (*post-test likelihood of a negative test*)?
- What would be the effect on the above values if the same test were applied to a population in which the disease was more or less prevalent?
- How *accurate* overall is the test (i.e. what proportion of test results correctly say whether the patient has or has not got the disease)?
- What is the *likelihood ratio* of a positive (or a negative) test (i.e. by how much does a positive (or negative) test increase (or decrease)the likelihood of the disease being present)?
- What, in summary, is the usefulness of this test in different groups and subgroups of patients?

SET ARTICLE

Piccinelli M, Tessari E, Bortolomasi M *et al.* Efficacy of the alcohol use disorders identification test as a screening tool for hazardous alcohol intake and related disorders in primary care: a validity study. *BMJ* 1997; **314**: 420–4.

Clinical scenario

A nurse practitioner in a large primary care centre runs a walk-in "well man" clinic. One patient, Mr Mario Pellento, is a 54-year-old Italian businessman. Mr Pellento arrives after the clinic has finished, smelling strongly of wine, and is rude to the receptionists. He is asked to return the following week for his check-up. The nurse wonders whether she might ask Mr Pellento a few questions next time to help decide whether he has alcohol dependence.

SUGGESTIONS FOR GROUP EXERCISES

When you have read the paper, try one or more of the following.
1. A teaching situation in which a group of students discusses the expressions "normal" and "abnormal" in relation to the results of diagnostic or screening tests.
2. A role play in which Mr Pellento is offered the screening questionnaire and, after completing it and scoring "positive", asks the meaning of the result.
3. A demonstration of how to calculate the likelihood ratio of this test, including (using role play if necessary) an explanation to someone who is confused about the meaning of this term.

SUGGESTION FOR INDIVIDUAL STUDY

Imagine you were the medical adviser to Mr Pellento's private health insurance company. He has passed on to you the fact that in the Alcohol Use Disorders Identification Test, he scored in the range indicating "harmful alcohol use". After completing the critical appraisal checklist for this article, compose a letter to the company's actuary, stating whether you would recommend increasing Mr Pellento's premiums for health insurance, send him for further tests or take no action. Justify this decision using arguments based on probabilities (i.e. Bayes' theorem).

		Result of gold standard test	
		Disease positive **a + c**	Disease negative **b + d**
Result of screening test	Test positive **a + b**	True positive **a**	False positive **b**
	c + d Test negative	**c** False negative	**d** True negative

Table 7.1 2×2 table notation for expressing the results of a validation study for a diagnostic or screening test

Feature of the test	Alternative name	Question which the feature addresses	Formula
Sensitivity	True positive rate (**P**ositive in **D**isease)	How good is this test at picking up people who have the condition?	a/a+c
Specificity	True negative rate (**N**egative in **H**ealth)	How good is this test at correctly excluding people without the condition?	d/b+d
Positive predictive value	Post-test probability of a positive test	If a person tests positive, what is the probability that (s)he has the condition?	a/a+b
Negative predictive value	Post-test probability of a negative test	If a person tests negative, what is the probability that (s)he does not have the condition?	d/c+d
Accuracy	–	What proportion of all tests have given the correct result (i.e. true positives and true negatives as a proportion of all results)?	a+d/a+b+c+d
Likelihood ratio of a positive test	–	How much more likely is positive test to be found in a person with, as opposed to without, the condition?	$\dfrac{\text{Sensitivity}}{(1-\text{specificity})}$

Table 7.2 Derivation of features of a diagnostic or screening test

CALCULATIONS

		Target disorder		Totals
		Present	Absent	
Diagnostic test result	Positive	a	b	a+b
	Negative	c	d	c+d
Totals		a+c	b+d	a+b+c+d

Sensitivity = a/(a+c)
Specificity = d/(b+d)
Prevalence in the study = (a+c)/(a+b+c+d)
Positive predictive value (in the study) = a/(a+b)
Negative predictive value (in the study) = d/(c+d)

FURTHER READING

Greenhalgh T. *How to read a paper: the basics of evidence based medicine*. London: BMJ Books, 1997. See in particular Chapter 4: Assessing methodological quality, pages 53–68 and Chapter 7: Papers that report diagnostic or screening tests, pages 97–110.

Jaeschke R, Guyatt G, Sackett DL. Users' guides to the medical literature. III. How to use an article about a diagnostic test. A. Are the results of the study valid? *JAMA* 1994; **271**: 389–91.

Jaeschke R, Guyatt G, Sackett DL. Users' guides to the medical literature. III. How to use an article about a diagnostic test. B. What were the results and will they help me in caring for my patients? *JAMA* 1994; **271**: 703–7.

CRITICAL APPRAISAL CHECKLIST FOR AN ARTICLE DESCRIBING A VALIDATION STUDY OF A SCREENING OR DIAGNOSTIC TEST

Note that the questions on the checklist are really looking for problems of bias, confounding, low power, and poor validity.

A. Are the results of the trial valid?	Yes/No/Don't know
1. Did the researchers make the diagnosis independently and blindly with both the test of interest, as well as a 'gold' standard (control) test?	
2. Was the test evaluated in people typical of patients you might expect to see in practice?	
3. Did the study contain enough cases to compare the new test and the gold standard test reliably? • Did the authors include a power calculation?	
4. Were *all* people diagnosed with both the test of interest as well as the 'gold' standard test (regardless of the results from either)?	
B. What are the results?	
5. Are the test's sensitivity and specificity good enough? • See table below; sensitivity should be high to catch as many cases as possible. Specificity should be high to rule out as many non-cases as possible.	
C. How relevant are the results?	
6. Is is possible to get a rough idea of how prevalent the condition you are trying to diagnose is in your patients (pre-test probability)?	
7. Is the diagnostic test likely to be accurate in your patients? • Would its predictive values be good enough for the prevalence of the condition in your patients? (See table below. Positive test results are more likely to be accurate when the condition is more common in people like your patient; negative test results are more likely to be accurate when the condition is less common in people like your patient.)	
8. Will the resulting positive and negative predictive values affect your management and help your patient? • Would the results change management? • Are patients willing to be treated?	
9. Is the test likely to be affordable, available, and acceptable in your setting?	

BMJ

Efficacy of the alcohol use disorders identification test as a screening tool for hazardous alcohol intake and related disorders in primary care: a validity study

Marco Piccinelli, *researcher*,[a] **Elisabetta Tessari**, *clinical psychologist*,[b] **Marco Bortolomasi**, *resident in psychiatry*,[b] **Orazio Piasere**, *resident in psychiatry*,[b] **Massimo Semenzin**, *resident in psychiatry*,[b] **Nicola Garzotto**, *associate professor of psychiatry*,[b] **Michele Tansella**, *professor of psychiatry*[a]

[a] Servizio di Psicologia Medica, Istituto di Psichiatria, Università di Verona, Verona, Italy,[b] Istituto di Psichiatria, Università di Verona, Verona, Italy

Correspondence to: Dr Marco Piccinelli Servizio di Psicologia Medica, Istituto di Psichiatria, Ospedale Policlinico, 37134 Verona, Italy (marpic@borgoroma.univr.it).

 Abstract

Objective: To determine the properties of the alcohol use disorders identification test in screening primary care attenders for alcohol problems.

Design: A validity study among consecutive primary care attenders aged 18-65 years. Every third subject completed the alcohol use disorders identification test (a 10 item self report questionnaire on alcohol intake and related problems) and was interviewed by an investigator with the composite international diagnostic interview alcohol use module (a standardised interview for the independent assessment of alcohol intake and related disorders).

Setting: 10 primary care clinics in Verona, north eastern Italy.

Patients: 500 subjects were approached and 482 (96.4%) completed evaluation.

Results: When the alcohol use disorders identification test was used to detect subjects with alcohol problems the area under the receiver operating characteristic curve was 0.95. The cut off score of 5 was associated with a sensitivity of 0.84, a specificity of 0.90, and a positive predictive value of 0.60. The screening ability of the total score derived from summing the responses to the five items minimising the probability of misclassification between subjects with and without alcohol problems provided an area under the receiver operating characteristic curve of 0.93. A score of 5 or more on the five items was associated with a sensitivity of 0.79, a specificity of 0.95, and a positive predictive value of 0.73.

Conclusions: The alcohol use disorders identification test performs well in detecting subjects with formal alcohol disorders and those with hazardous alcohol intake. Using five of the 10 items on the questionnaire gives reasonable accuracy, and these are recommended as questions of choice to screen patients for alcohol problems.

Originally published in *BMJ* 1997; **314**: 420–4.

Introduction

Hazardous alcohol intake and related disorders are a major public health issue. Data from the World Health Organisation's collaborative project on psychological problems in general health care have shown that alcohol dependence or harmful use of alcohol as defined by the 10th revision of the International Classification of Diseases (ICD-10) is present in about 6% of primary care attenders, ranking third in frequency after major depression and generalised anxiety.[1]

In addition to formal alcohol disorders such as dependence or harmful use, increasing attention has been paid to hazardous alcohol intake, defined as a level of consumption or pattern of drinking which, if it persists, is likely to result in harm. Hazardous alcohol intake is directly or indirectly implicated in many physical, psychological, and social problems, imposing a substantial financial burden on the drinkers and on society.[2][3][4] Moreover, drinking at levels causing detectable biochemical abnormalities is associated with a mortality that is twice that of the normal population.[5]

Primary prevention often requires national strategies promoting an overall decrease of alcohol consumption in the population. By contrast, secondary prevention can effectively be undertaken at the primary care level by means of early detection of people with hazardous alcohol intake and time limited interventions aimed at decreasing alcohol consumption and thus the likelihood of subsequent harm and dependence. Though several screening instruments have been developed that are fairly short and easy to administer, they tend to detect severe alcohol disorders such as dependence and overlook hazardous drinking. The WHO therefore devised a 10 item questionnaire–the alcohol use disorders identification test[6]–whose distinct advantage is the ability to detect both formal alcohol disorders and hazardous alcohol intake.

We investigated the screening properties of the alcohol use disorders identification test in the detection of primary care attenders with formal alcohol disorders or hazardous alcohol intake.

 ## Subjects and method

Sampling strategy

Ten primary care physicians in Verona, north eastern Italy, allowed investigators to visit their clinics twice a week, once in the morning and once in the afternoon. Among patients aged 18-65 attending other than for a prescription, every third patient was approached up to a total of 50 patients at each clinic. Subjects were informed about the project and told that responses would be kept confidential. Those agreeing to participate had the size of a standard drink[7] explained to them (see box) and then completed the alcohol use disorders identification test in the waiting room. In addition, the alcohol use module of the composite international diagnostic interview[8][9] was administered by an investigator at the clinic on the same day or at the patient's home within a week. Investigators included three doctors and a final year student in psychology; they received group training in administering the composite international diagnostic interview and practised individually in role play sessions before the fieldwork. Finally, for each eligible subject the primary care physician rated on a form a list of clinical signs often related to alcohol consumption (for example, abnormal skin vascularisation, jaundice, hand tremor, liver characteristics); noted drinking behaviour over the previous 12 months (no alcohol abuse, occasional alcohol abuse, regular alcohol abuse); and noted the intake of psychotropic drugs during the two weeks before examination.

Instruments

The alcohol use disorders identification test is a self administered questionnaire including three items on the amount and frequency of drinking, three on alcohol dependence, and four on common problems caused by alcohol (see 3). Each item is scored 0-4, giving a total score of 40.

The composite international diagnostic interview is a standardised diagnostic interview for assessing mental disorders according to criteria of the ICD-10[10] and the *Diagnostic and Statistical Manual of Mental Disorders, Third Edition, Revised* (DSM-III-R).[11]

English versions of both instruments were translated into Italian, and the Italian versions were independently translated back into English; changes were made where necessary in order to ensure close correspondence between the original and Italian versions.

Diagnostic criteria

The screening properties of the alcohol use disorders identification test were tested against the standard criteria listed in the box. Criteria were fulfilled during the 12 months before examination and based on responses to the alcohol use module of the composite international diagnostic interview, which was the standard for the study.

Alcohol dependence and harmful use were diagnosed according to ICD-10 criteria. Defining hazardous alcohol intake was difficult, as the risk associated with alcohol consumption lies along a continuum. Recommendations on levels of safe drinking published in the United Kingdom by the Health Education Authority and supported by the Royal College of Psychiatrists, the Royal College of General Practitioners, and the Royal College of Physicians[12][13] suggest that 30 g pure ethanol daily in men and 20 g daily in women constitute hazardous alcohol intake. The definitions of hazardous alcohol intake in this study (see box), based on categories of quantity and frequency of alcohol consumption from the alcohol use module of the composite international diagnostic interview, closely corresponded to the recommendations reported above.

Statistics

The screening properties of the alcohol use disorders indentifcation test were investigated by receiver operating characteristic analysis. This technique summarises the validity coefficients of a test and provides an overall index of diagnostic accuracy (that is, the area under the receiver operating characteristic curve) by plotting sensitivity against the false positive rate for all possible cut off scores. An area under the receiver operating characteristic curve of 0.5 is obtained when the discriminatory ability of a test is no better than chance; a value of 1.0 represents perfect discriminatory ability.[14]
A computer program for receiver operating characteristic analysis similar to that developed by Dorfman and Alf[15] and modified by Metz et al[16] was used in this study.

> **Standard diagnostic criteria used in validating alcohol use disorders identification test**
>
> **Alcohol dependence (at least three items required)(ICD-10)**
>
> 1. Strong desire or sense of compulsion to take the substance
>
> 2. Impaired capacity to control substance taking behaviour in terms of onset, termination, or levels of use
>
> 3. Physiological withdrawal state when substance use is reduced or stopped or use of the substance to relieve or avoid withdrawal symptoms
>
> 4. Evidence of tolerance to the effects of the substance
>
> 5. Other pleasures or interests being given up or reduced because of the substance use
>
> 6. Persistent substance use despite clear evidence of harmful consequences
>
> **Harmful alcohol use (ICD-10)**
>
> (a) Clear evidence that the substance use is responsible for (or is substantially contributing to) physical or psychological harm
>
> (b) The nature of the harm is clearly identifiable and specified
>
> (c) The pattern of use has persisted for at least one month or has occurred repeatedly within the 12 month period
>
> (d) The subject does not fulfil criteria for alcohol dependence
>
> **Hazardous alcohol intake**
>
> *Men:* Three to seven drinks almost every day or seven or more drinks at least three times a week
>
> *Women:* Two to five drinks almost every day or five or more drinks at least three times a week
>
> *A standard drink* was defined as equivalent volumes containing an average of 13.5 g ethanol. Definitions of a standard drink were based on local alcoholic beverages and included one glass of wine (125 ml), one bottle of beer (500 ml), and one measure of spirits (40 ml)[7]

Logistic regression analysis was performed to identify linear combinations of items in the alcohol use disorders identification test that minimised the probability of misclassification between subjects with and without alcohol dependence, harmful use, or hazardous intake. A stepwise selection of predictor variables was adopted by using the likelihood ratio statistic as a test for removal and a probability level of 0.10 to remove a variable.

▶ Results

Five hundred subjects were approached at the primary care clinics, of whom 489 (97.8%) agreed to participate and 482 (96.4%) completed the evaluation. Most were women (n=306; 63.5%), married (290; 60.2%), and employed (274; 56.8%) and had low educational attainment (320 (66.4%) educated to secondary school level only). Mean age was 42.2 (SD 14.4) years. Seven subjects (1.5%) fulfilled ICD-10 criteria for alcohol dependence; all were men, with a median age of 43 years (range 21–61 years). Fifteen subjects (3.1%) fulfilled ICD-10 criteria for harmful alcohol use; 13 (86.7%) were men, with a median age of 50 years (range 24–65 years).Lastly, 62 subjects (12.9%) satisfied criteria for hazardous alcohol intake; 51 (82.3%) were men, with a median age of 48 years (range 21–65 years).

The screening characteristics of the alcohol use disorders identification test were initially tested separately against the diagnostic criteria listed in the box. The questionnaire performed well in detecting subjects with alcohol dependence (area under receiver operating characteristic curve 0.91; 95% confidence interval 0.88 to 0.94), harmful alcohol use (0.90; 0.88 to 0.92), and hazardous alcohol intake (0.92; 0.90 to 0.93). However, though sensitivity and specificity were above 0.8 irrespective of the criterion used, positive predictive values (that is, the probability of having the disorder among patients with positive test results) were low, indicating a high proportion of false positive results.

As the alcohol use disorders identification test is expected to be more suitable for initial screening of people with probable alcohol problems of any type rather than for accurate detection of people with formal alcohol disorders, the screening characteristics of the questionnaire were tested against all three drinking categories considered together. Table 1 shows that the performance of the questionnaire was high, with an area under the receiver operating characteristic curve of about 0.95. The cut off score of 5 provided a good trade off between sensitivity (0.84) and specificity (0.90); however, the positive predictive value was comparatively low, indicating that 40% of subjects scoring 5 or higher were false positive cases. Higher positive predictive values were found at higher cut off scores, though at the expense of decreased sensitivity; higher positive predictive values might be expected at lower cut off scores in populations with a higher prevalence of alcohol problems.

Table 1 Validity coefficents of 10 item alcohol use disorders identification test in detection of subjects with and without alcohol dependence, harmful alcohol use, or hazardous alcohol intake considered together

Cut off	Sensitivity	Specificity	Positive predictive value†	Positive predictive value 25%‡	Positive predictive value 50%§
≥1	1.00	0.27	0.19	0.25	0.41
≥3	0.96	0.58	0.28	0.36	0.53
≥5	0.84	0.90	0.60	0.68	0.81
≥7	0.54	0.97	0.73	0.80	0.89
≥9	0.43	0.99	0.86	0.90	0.95
≥11	0.31	1.00	1.00	1.00	1.00

Area under receiver operating characteristic curve 0.949 (95% confidence interval 0.940 to 0.959).
†Positive predictive value in study sample (prevalence of alcohol dependence, harmful use, or hazardous intake 14.5%).
‡Represents positive predictive value when prevalence of alcohol dependence, harmful use, or hazardous intake in population is 25%.
§Represents positive predictive value when prevalence of alcohol dependence, harmful use, or hazardous intake in population is 50%.

As low positive predictive values might result from the 10 items of the questionnaire being given the same weight in computing a total score, logistic regression analysis was performed to identify the items minimising the probability of misclassification between subjects with and without alcohol dependence, harmful use, or hazardous intake considered together. Estimated coefficients and related statistics from logistic regression analysis are not reported here but are available on request. Five items were retained in the model (goodness of fit 556.5; df=463, P=0.002): item 1 (frequency of drinking), item 2 (number of drinks on a typical day), item 4 (unable to stop drinking), item 5 (failing to do what was normally expected), and item 10 (another person concerned about subject's drinking or suggesting that it should be cut down). The discriminatory ability of the total score resulting from summing the responses to the five items is shown in table 2. Overall performance was high, with an area under the receiver operating characteristic curve of 0.93. A total score of 5 or more on the five selected items was associated with a sensitivity of 0.79, a specificity of 0.95, and a positive predictive value of 0.73; moreover, the probability of a subject scoring less than 5 having alcohol problems was less than 4%.

Table 2 Validity coefficients of five items of alcohol use disorders identification test selected through logistic regression analysis in detection of subjects with and without alcohol dependence, harmful alcohol use, or hazardous alcohol intake considered together

Cut off	Sensitivity	Specificity	Positive predictive value†	Positive predictive value 25%‡	Positive predictive value 50%§
≥1	1.00	0.27	0.19	0.25	0.41
≥3	0.96	0.58	0.28	0.36	0.53
≥5	0.84	0.90	0.60	0.68	0.81
≥7	0.54	0.97	0.73	0.80	0.89
≥9	0.43	0.99	0.86	0.90	0.95

Area under receiver operating characteristic curve 0.949 (95% confidence interval 0.940 to 0.959).
†Positive predictive value in study sample (prevalence of alcohol dependence, harmful use, or hazardous intake 14.5%).
‡Represents positive predictive value when prevalence of alcohol dependence, harmful use, or hazardous intake in population is 25%.
§Represents positive predictive value when prevalence of alcohol dependence, harmful use, or hazardous intake in population is 50%.

These findings can be compared with the low ability of doctors to detect patients with hazardous alcohol intake or formal alcohol disorders, only 39% of these patients being rated as abusers of alcohol either occasionally or regularly.

 ## Discussion

This study shows that the alcohol use disorders identification test is a simple questionnaire that takes only a few minutes to complete and performs well in detecting both people with formal alcohol disorders and those with hazardous alcohol intake. As five of the 10 items on the questionnaire are reasonably accurate for screening, physicians or other primary care professionals are recommended to use them as questions of choice to screen patients for alcohol problems of any type. Subsequent detailed evaluation can then be offered to those with positive test results in order to reach firm diagnostic conclusions. Our findings are similar to those from the exploratory WHO multicentre study,[17] in which the 10 item alcohol use disorders identification test had a mean sensitivity of 0.80 and a mean specificity of 0.89 across participating centres.

Several screening instruments for alcohol disorders have been tested, including the Michigan alcoholism screening test[18] and its shorter versions[19 20 21], the CAGE questionnaire,[22] the Veterans alcoholism screening test,[23] and the primary care evaluation of mental disorders.[24] In general the ability of these instruments to detect formal alcohol disorders is comparable to that of the alcohol use disorders identification test.[24 25] However, most of the instruments have not been tested in the detection of hazardous alcohol intake; when this was done sensitivity failed at unacceptable levels.[26] Other instruments, such as the Munich alcoholism test,[27] require clinical examination to elicit physical signs related to excessive alcohol consumption, which makes them less likely to be used by busy physicians or prevents their use by non-medical professionals. Hence the alcohol use disorders identification test has definite advantages over existing screening instruments, as it can screen both for hazardous alcohol intake (possibly in patients before symptoms begin or in those with mild symptoms) and for formal alcohol disorders and can be used by health workers with no formal medical training.

We acknowledge that our study has possible limitations. Firstly, as data on alcohol consumption in the area were not available we did not perform a power calculation for required sample size and selecting comparatively few patients with alcohol problems might have affected the findings. Secondly, a proportion of subjects with alcohol problems might be expected to underreport them both on the alcohol use disorders identification test and at the diagnostic interview, with validity coefficients of the questionnaire being artificially raised. Independent data provided by primary care physicians suggest that this bias was limited, as three quarters of subjects with physical signs possibly due to excessive drinking reported alcohol problems at interview. No other sources of information (for example, spouse or other key informants, hospital records, biological markers, etc) were available to examine this issue further. Finally, some items included in the alcohol use disorders identification test were embodied within standard validating criteria, which might also have resulted in inflated estimates of test accuracy. Other validity studies using different sources of information and standard criteria may be useful to clarify this issue.

Acknowledgements

We thank the following primary care physicians for collaborating: M Bagnani, A Battagia, F Boninsegna, G Dal Cortivo, G Insom, R Montolli, G Piubello, G V Romanelli, P Sandri, and L Serra. We are also grateful to Dr Giulia Bisoffi for commenting on the study design.

Funding: None.

Conflict of interest: None.

Appendix

Alcohol use disorders indentification test. (Scores for response categories are given in parentheses)

1   *How often do you have a drink containing alcohol?*
    (0) Never   (1) Monthly or   (2) Two to four   (3) Two or three   (4) Four or more
                     less   times a month   times a week   times a week

2   *How many drinks containing alcohol do you have on a typical day when you are drinking?*
    (0) 1 or 2   (1) 3 or 4   (2) 5 or 6   (3) 7 to 9   (4) 10 or more

3   *How often do you have six or more drinks on one occasion?*
    (0) Never   (1) Less than   (2) Monthly   (3) Weekly   (4) Daily or
                     monthly   almost daily

4   *How often during the past year have you found that you were not able to stop drinking once you have started?*
    (0) Never   (1) Less than   (2) Monthly   (3) Weekly   (4) Daily or
                     monthly   almost daily

5 *How often during the past year have you failed to do what was normally expected of you because of drinking?*
(0) Never (1) Less than (2) Monthly (3) Weekly (4) Daily or
      monthly   almost daily

6 *How often during the past year have you needed a first drink in the morning to get yourself going after a heavy drinking session?*
(0) Never (1) Less than (2) Monthly (3) Weekly (4) Daily or
      monthly   almost daily

7 *How often during the past year have you had a feeling of guilt or remorse after drinking?*
(0) Never (1) Less than (2) Monthly (3) Weekly (4) Daily or
      monthly   almost daily

8 *How often during the past year have you been unable to remember what happened the night before because you had been drinking?*
(0) Never (1) Less than (2) Monthly (3) Weekly (4) Daily or
      monthly   almost daily

9 *Have you or has someone else been injured as a result of your drinking?*
(0) No (2) Yes, but not in the past year (4) Yes, during the past year

10 *Has a relative or friend or a doctor or other health worker been concerned about your drinking or suggested you cut down?*
(0) No (2) Yes, but not in the past year (4) Yes, during the past year

References

1. Goldberg D, Lecrubier Y. Forms and frequency of mental disorders across centres. In: Üstün TB, Sartorius N, eds. *Mental illness in general health care. An international study.* New York: John Wiley & Sons, 1995:324–34.
2. Her Majesty's Stationery Office. *Lord President's report on action against alcohol misuse.* London: HMSO, 1991.
3. Rice DP, Kelman S, Miller LS. Estimates of economic costs of alcohol and drug abuse and mental illness, 1985 and 1988. *Public Health Rep* 1991;**106**:280–92.
4. Nakamura K, Tanaka A, Takano T. The social cost of alcohol abuse in Japan. *J Stud Alcohol* 1993;**54**:618–25.
5. Anderson P. *Management of drinking problems* . Copenhagen: WHO Regional Publications, 1990:44–6. (European series No 32.)
6. Babor TF, de la Fuente JR, Saunders J, Grant M. *The alcohol use disorders identification test. Guidelines for use in primary health care.* Geneva: World Health Organisation, 1989.
7. Modonutti G. Studio multicentrico sui modelli di consumo delle bevande alcoliche espressi dalla popolazione generale. In: Allamani A, Cipriani F, Orlandini D, eds. *Alcologia in Italia. Una prospettiva epidemiologica.* Bologna: Editrice Compositori Bologna, 1993:**51**.
8. Robins LN, Wing JK, Wittchen HU, Helzer JE, Babor TF, Burke J, *et al* . The composite international diagnostic interview. An epidemiologic instrument. *Arch Gen Psychiatry* 1988;**45**:1069–77.
9. World Health Organisation. *CIDI–core. Composite international diagnostic interview, core version.* Geneva: World Health Organisation, 1990.
10. World Health Organisation. *International classification of diseases. 10th Revision* . Geneva: WHO, 1992.
11. American Psychiatric Association. *Diagnostic and statistical manual of mental disorders, third edition, revised.* Washington, DC: APA, 1987.
12. Catarino PA. Is there a safe level of drinking? A student's view. *Alcohol Alcohol* 1992;**27**:465–70.
13. Government review of the sensible drinking message: a Medical Council on Alcoholism view. Do not change the numbers–clarify the message. *Alcohol Alcohol* 1995;**30**:571–5.

14. Rey JM, Morris-Yates A, Stanislaw H. Measuring the accuracy of diagnostic tests using receiver operating characteristics (ROC) analysis. *Int J Methods Psychiatr Res* 1992;**2**:39–50.
15. Dorfman D, Alf E. Maximum-likelihood estimation of parameters of signal detection theory and determination of confidence intervals: rating method data. *J Math Psychol* 1966;**6**:487–96.
16. Metz CE, Wang PL, Kronman HB. *ROCFIT.* Chicago: Department of Radiology and the Franklin McLean Memorial Research Institute, University of Chicago, 1984.
17. Saunders JB, Aasland OG. *WHO collaborative project on identification and treatment of persons with harmful alcohol consumption. Report on phase I: development of a screening instrument.* Geneva: World Health Organisation, 1987.
18. Selzer ML. The Michigan alcoholism screening test. The quest for a new diagnostic instrument. *Am J Psychiatry* 1971;**127**:1653–8.
19. Pokorny AD, Miller BA, Kaplan HB. The brief MAST. A shortened version of the Michigan alcoholism screening test. *Am J Psychiatry* 1972;**129**:342–5.
20. Selzer ML, Vinokur A, Van Roojen LA. A self-administered short Michigan alcoholism screening test (SMAST). *J Stud Alcohol* 1975;**36**:117–26.
21. Kristenson H, Trell E. Indicators of alcohol consumption. Comparison between a questionnaire (Mm-MAST), interviews and serum gamma-glutamyl transferase (GGT) in a health survey of middle-aged males. *Br J Addict* 1982;**77**:297–304.
22. Mayfield D, McLeod G, Hall P. The CAGE questionnaire. Validation of a new alcoholism screening test. *Am J Psychiatry* 1974;**131**:1121–3.
23. Magruder-Habib K, Harris KE, Fraker GG. Validation of the Veterans alcoholism screening test. *J Stud Alcohol* 1982;**43**:910–26.
24. Spitzer RL, Williams JBW, Kroenke K, Linzer M, Verloin deGruy III F, Hahn SR, *et al.* Utility of a new procedure for diagnosing mental disorders in primary care. The PRIME-MD study. *JAMA* 1994;**272**:1749–56.
25. Magruder-Habib K, Stevens HA, Alling WC. Relative performance of the MAST, VAST, and CAGE versus DSM-III-R criteria for alcohol dependence. *J Clin Epidemiol* 1993;**46**:435–41.
26. Kitchens JM. Does this patient have an alcohol problem? *JAMA* 1994;**272**:1782–7.
27. Feuerlein W, Ringer C, Kufner H, Antons K. The diagnosis of alcoholism–the Munich alcoholism test (MALT). *Int J Rehabil Res* 1979;**2**:533–4.

(Accepted 6 December 1996)

Papers that summarise other papers (systematic review and meta-analysis)

BACKGROUND

The "gold standard" in clinical evidence for most types of research questions is the systematic review of original research trials, with numerical meta-analysis if appropriate. But systematic reviews can themselves be done well or badly. One defining feature of a systematic review is the presence of a methods section that allows the critical reader to assess how far the authors have achieved the goal of rigorous secondary research.

SUGGESTED AIM FOR THIS SESSION

For participants to master, and become confident in helping others to master, the ability to evaluate an article on systematic review or meta-analysis and decide whether it applies in particular clinical circumstances.

SUGGESTED LEARNING OBJECTIVES FOR THIS SESSION

By the end of this session, participants should be able to evaluate a published article describing an overview of original research studies and in particular to:
● decide whether the clinical question addressed by an overview is appropriate and sufficiently focused;
● determine whether the results are valid, i.e. whether the methods used for the review were sufficiently reliable and well conducted;
● interpret the quantitative findings in the results;
● decide whether the conclusions are justified;
● relate the results and conclusions to their own clinical practice.

SET ARTICLE

Gotzsche PC, Hammarquist C, Burr M. House dust mite control measures in the management of asthma: meta-analysis. *BMJ* 1998; **317**: 1105–10.

ADDITIONAL REPRINT

Davey SG, Egger M. Meta-analysis. Unresolved issues and future developments. *BMJ* 1998; **316**: 221–5.

Clinical scenario

Johnny Brown is a 3-year-old boy who has recently developed moderate asthma. He is treated with prophylactic inhaled steroids but remains poorly controlled. Skin prick testing confirms sensitivity to house dust mite. Johnny's parents are advised to adopt radical measures to eradicate dust from their home. They remove all rugs and feather bedding, purchase a new high-suction vacuum cleaner, and clean the house regularly with an antimite chemical cleaner. Altogether they estimate that they have invested several hundred pounds in the measures to eradicate the allergen but Johnny's asthma is no better. Mrs Brown surfs the Internet for information from professional sources and finds the paper reprinted below on house dust mite control measures. She asks her GP to help her interpret it.

SUGGESTIONS FOR GROUP EXERCISES

When you have read the paper, try one or more of the following.
1. A role play of a consultation in which one member of your group represents Mrs Brown and another represents her GP.
2. A role play of an interview between a lay member of the National Asthma Campaign and a salesman from a company that makes anti-house dust mite vacuum cleaners, facilitated by a health professional with a knowledge of evidence-based health care and copies of the relevant paper.
3. A teaching situation in which a mixed group of paediatric asthma nurses and senior house officers are asked to appraise the paper.

SUGGESTION FOR INDIVIDUAL STUDY

Consider the second of the above group exercises. Imagine you are a medical journalist approached by a person with asthma who tells you of this encounter. Write a short newspaper article giving your opinion on the salesman's claim that the vacuum cleaner is a good investment.

FURTHER READING

Chalmers I, Sackett D, Silagy C. The Cochrane Collaboration. In: Maynard A, Chalmers I, eds. *Non-random reflections on health services research.* London: BMJ Books 1997: 231–9.

Greenhalgh T. *How to read a paper: the basics of evidence-based medicine.* London: BMJ Books, 1997. See in particular Chapter 8: Papers that summarise other papers, pages 111–27.

Oxman AD, Cook DJ, Guyatt GH. Users' guides to the medical literature. VI. How to use an overview. *JAMA* 1994; **272**: 1367–71.

CRITICAL APPRAISAL CHECKLIST FOR AN ARTICLE DESCRIBING A SYSTEMATIC REVIEW

Note that the questions on the checklist are really looking for problems of bias, confounding, low power, and poor validity.

A. Was selection of studies valid?	Yes/No/Don't know
1. Did the trial address a clearly focused question Clearly defined: • Population • Intervention • Outcome(s)	
2. Were high-quality, relevant studies included? • Robust study design (RCTs?) • Sufficient sample size (power)? • Addressing relevant question (population/intervention/ outcome)?	
3. Is it unlikely that important, relevant studies were missed? • Repeatable search strategy? • Comprehensive search strategy, including relevant databases *and* other, unpublished sources for information (e.g. EMBASE, Cochrane Library controlled trials register, MEDLINE back to 1966, contacts from reference lists)?	
4. Was the validity of the included studies assessed properly? • Reproducible (explicit) assessment method? • More than one independent assessor?	
5. Were the results similar from study to study (i.e. were they comparable)?	
B. What are the results?	
6. What are the overall results of the review?	
7. How precise were the results (e.g. measures of risk, confidence intervals, p-values)?	
8. Can the results be applied to my patients? (Compare patient with review population, intervention, outcome)	
C. How relevant are the results to me?	
9. Were sufficient important outcomes (for me) considered?	

House dust mite control measures in the management of asthma: meta-analysis

Peter C Gøtzsche, Cecilia Hammarquist, Michael Burr

Abstract

Objective To determine whether patients with asthma who are sensitive to mites benefit from measures designed to reduce their exposure to house dust mite antigen in the home.

Design Meta-analysis of randomised trials that investigated the effects on asthma patients of chemical or physical measures to control mites, or both, in comparison with an untreated control group. All trials in any language were eligible for inclusion.

Subjects Patients with bronchial asthma as diagnosed by a doctor and sensitisation to mites as determined by skin prick testing, bronchial provocation testing, or serum assays for specific IgE antibodies.

Main outcome measures Number of patients whose allergic symptoms improved, improvement in asthma symptoms, improvement in peak expiratory flow rate. Outcomes measured on different scales were combined using the standardised effect size method (the difference in effect was divided by the standard deviation of the measurements).

Results 23 studies were included in the meta-analysis; 6 studies used chemical methods to reduce exposure to mites, 13 used physical methods, and 4 used a combination. Altogether, 41/113 patients exposed to treatment interventions improved compared with 38/117 in the control groups (odds ratio 1.20, 95% confidence interval 0.66 to 2.18). The standardised mean difference for improvement in asthma symptoms was -0.06 (95% confidence interval -0.54 to 0.41). For peak flow rate measured in the morning the standardised mean difference was -0.03 (-0.25 to 0.19). As measured in the original units this difference between the treatment and the control group corresponds to -3 l/min (95% confidence interval -25 l/min to 19 l/min). The results were similar in the subgroups of trials that reported successful reduction in exposure to mites or had long follow up times.

Conclusion Current chemical and physical methods aimed at reducing exposure to allergens from house dust mites seem to be ineffective and cannot be recommended as prophylactic treatment for asthma patients sensitive to mites.

Introduction

The major allergen in house dust is derived from mites, and a recent review concluded that the environmental control of allergens should be an integral part of the management of sensitised patients.[1] Some of the evidence in the review, however, was derived from observational studies. Since clinical trials have shown equivocal results of the effectiveness of measures to reduce exposure to mite antigen, we decided to synthesise the findings of all clinical trials.

Methods

Our objective was to determine whether patients with asthma who were sensitised to house dust mites benefited from measures designed to reduce their exposure to mite antigen in the home. All randomised trials in any language performed at any time that compared chemical (acaricidal) or physical measures (such as vacuum cleaning, heating, barrier methods, or air filtration systems) to control mites and analysed their effects on patients with bronchial asthma as compared with an untreated control group were eligible for inclusion in the meta-analysis. Asthma had to have been diagnosed by a doctor and sensitisation to mites had to have been assessed by skin tests, bronchial provocation tests, or serum assays for specific IgE antibodies.

Search strategy

We searched the Asthma and Wheez* databases set up by the Cochrane Airways Group which contain records from the Cumulative Index to Nursing and Allied Health Literature, Medline, and Embase. Mite* in the title, abstract, or keyword (descriptor) field was combined with random*, trial*, placebo, double-blind, double blind, single-blind, single blind, comparative study, or controlled study in all fields. Primary authors were contacted to obtain additional information if necessary. CH searched issues of *Respiration* (1980-96) and MB searched *Clinical and Experimental Allergy* (1980-96) by hand.

Extraction of data

Two of the authors (CH and MB) selected the trials for inclusion. Two (PCG and CH) extracted data on the following outcomes: subjective wellbeing, improvement in asthma symptoms, use of drugs to control asthma, number of days of sick leave taken from school or work, number of unscheduled visits made to a doctor or hospital, forced expiratory volume in 1 second,

Editorial
by Strachan

Nordic Cochrane Centre, Rigshospitalet, Department 7112, DK-2200 Copenhagen N, Denmark
Peter C Gøtzsche, *director*

Executive Office, Unit of Public Health, Municipality of Gotland, S-62181 Visby, Sweden
Cecilia Hammarquist, *director*

Centre for Applied Public Health Medicine, University of Wales College of Medicine, Cardiff CF1 3NW
Michael Burr, *consultant*

Correspondence to:
Dr Gøtzsche
p.c.gotzsche@
cochrane.dk

BMJ 1998;317:1105–10

Originally published in *BMJ* 1998; **317**: 1105–1110.

Characteristics of the 23 studies included in the meta-analysis of methods to control exposure to mites among asthma patients

Study (year)	Type of intervention	Design	Mean age or age range of patients (years)	No of patients in study	No of patients not completing study	Length of follow up	Reduction in exposure to mites or mite antigen achieved
Dietemann et al (1993)[9]	Chemical	Parallel trial, double blind	36	26	3	1 year	No
Ehnert et al (1992)[11]	Chemical	Parallel trial, double blind	10	16	0	1 year	No
Geller-Bernstein et al (1995)[12]	Chemical	Parallel trial, double blind	9	35	3	6 months	No
Van der Heide et al (1997)[24]	Chemical	Parallel trial, double blind	31	40	0	1 year	No
Reiser et al (1990)[16]	Chemical	Parallel trial, double blind	5-16	51	5	3 months	No
Sette et al (1994)[17]	Chemical	Parallel trial, double blind	13	24	0	2 weeks	No
Antonicelli et al (1991)[5]	Physical	Crossover trial, assessor blind	16	9	0	8 weeks	No
Burr et al (1976)[6]	Physical	Crossover trial, no blinding	33	32	0	6 weeks	NA
Burr et al (1980)[7]	Physical	Parallel trial, double blind	9	55	2	8 weeks	No
Burr et al (1980)[8]	Physical	Crossover trial, no blinding	9	21	0	1 month	No
Gillies et al (1987)[13]	Physical	Parallel trial, no blinding	10	26	1	6 weeks	No
Huss et al (1992)[25]	Physical	Parallel trial, no blinding	44	52	0	12 weeks	Yes
Maesen et al (1977)[26]	Physical	Crossover trial, double blind	7-55	30	2	1 month	NA
Mitchell and Elliott (1980)[15]	Physical	Crossover trial, no blinding	10	10	0	4 weeks	NA
Verrall et al (1988)[18]	Physical	Crossover trial, double blind	14	16	3	3 weeks	NA
Walshaw and Evans (1986)[19]	Physical	Parallel trial, no blinding	34	50	8	1 year	Yes
Warburton et al (1994)[20]	Physical	Crossover trial, double blind	46	13	1	4 weeks	No
Warner et al (1993)[21]	Physical	Crossover trial, double blind	9	20	6	6 weeks	Yes
Zwemer and Karibo (1973)[22]	Physical	Crossover trial, double blind	6-16	18	6	4 weeks	NA
Carswell et al (1996)[23]	Combination	Parallel trial, double blind	10	70	21	24 weeks	Yes
Dorward et al (1988)[10]	Combination	Parallel trial, assessor blind	25	21	3	8 weeks	Yes
Ehnert et al (1992)[11]	Combination	Parallel trial, no blinding	10	16	0	1 year	Yes
Marks et al (1994)[14]	Combination	Parallel trial, participants blind	35	35	5	6 months	No

NA=not assessed.

peak expiratory flow rate, provocative concentration that causes a 20% fall in forced expiratory volume in 1 second, and results of skin prick testing. Ambiguities were resolved by discussion.

Statistical methods

Review Manager software was used to analyse the data.[2] If $P < 0.10$ in the test for heterogeneity a random effects analysis was carried out. Since the results from crossover trials were usually reported as if they had come from a parallel group trial we used the data accordingly and assumed that no carryover effect had occurred. Continuous data were often presented on different scales in different studies (for example, peak expiratory flow rate was given either as absolute values or as a per cent of predicted values). Because of this, we calculated the standardised mean difference in our analysis of these data. With this method, the difference in effect is divided by the standard deviation of the measurements. Since data on wellbeing and improvements in asthma symptoms were closely related we summarised categorical data as the number of patients whose asthma improved; we summarised continuous data in the category of asthma symptoms. In general, the provocative concentration that causes a 20% fall in the forced expiratory volume in 1 second had been analysed after logarithmic transformation because the data were highly skewed. If the mean values and standard deviations had been converted from the logarithmic to the arithmetic scale we reconverted them.[3] We excluded data on the provocative concentration from one study which had not used logarithmic transformation (see appendix 1 on the website).

In studies in which the use of several anti-asthma treatments had been reported we used the data on bronchodilators. In studies in which data were recorded at several points in time we used the longest observation period during which patients were still on randomised treatment.

We did not adjust for baseline differences since inequalities occurring despite randomisation would be expected to cancel each other out over a number of trials. Furthermore, baseline values were not always available. If we had made adjustments when possible we would have risked biasing the review since investigators may be inclined to show baseline differences and adjust for them when this procedure favours the experimental treatment. Bias occurring during the analysis of data is common and almost always favours the new treatment.[4]

Results

Trials included in the analysis

Altogether, 458 references were identified; half of these were irrelevant and the other half were retrieved so that the full study could be examined. Eighteen of the 229 studies met the inclusion criteria.[5-22] Another four trials were retrieved from MB's personal archive.[23-26] The reference lists of the 229 articles retrieved were also searched but no further appropriate studies were found. One of the papers included in the analysis[11] reported on a trial with three arms; this was treated as two separate trials in the meta-analysis. Thus, most of the analyses below refer to 23 trials. (A list of the excluded trials which were not evidently irrelevant and the reasons for their exclusion appear in appendix 2 on the website.)

All studies had used skin prick testing for diagnosis of mite sensitisation. Extracts were from *Dermatophagoides pteronyssinus* or *D farinae* except in two trials which had used an unspecified extract of house dust.[22 26] Two trials also used a serum assay for specific IgE antibodies.[9 11] Patients had mostly been recruited

115

from asthma and chest clinics. The specific criteria for the diagnosis of asthma were mentioned only in four papers.[11 14 17 25]

Six studies used chemical methods to reduce exposure to mites,[9 11 12 16 17 24] 13 used physical methods,[5-8 13 15 18-22 25 26] and four used a combination of methods.[10 11 14 23] Five studies did not assess the reduction of the population of mites.[6 15 18 22 26] Reduction in the exposure to mites occurred in six studies[10 19 21 23 25]; reduction was unsuccessful in 12.[5 7-9 11-14 16 17 20 24] The length of follow up, from two weeks to one year, and other characteristics of the studies are shown in the table.

Only one study reported enough information to allow us to determine that allocation had been adequately concealed[12]; in the remaining articles authors stated that the study was randomised. Thirteen of the studies were double blind or placebo controlled with blind assessment; two studies used blinded assessors and one had blinded participants; nine were crossover studies (table). Altogether, 686 patients were enrolled in the studies.

Results of meta-analysis
The total number of patients who improved after intervention was similar to the total number who improved among the control groups (41/113 in treatment group v 38/117 in control group, odds ratio 1.20, 95% confidence interval 0.66 to 2.18) (fig 1). Improvements in asthma symptoms were heterogeneous (P<0.0001) but there was no indication of an effect. The standardised mean difference of these scores was −0.06 (95% confidence interval −0.54 to 0.41) (fig 2). The result was similar when analysis was done with a fixed effects model (−0.01, −0.28 to 0.26).

The most commonly reported outcome was peak expiratory flow rate in the morning (fig 3). The time of

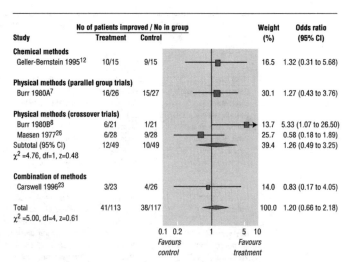

Fig 1 Odds ratios (95% confidence interval) of number of asthma patients whose symptoms improved after the use of either chemical or physical methods to reduce exposure to house dust mites

day that peak expiratory flow was measured was not stated in one study[19]; we assumed that it had been measured in the morning. The standardised mean difference between peak expiratory flow rates was −0.03 (−0.25 to 0.19). In the analysis of chemical methods to reduce the population of house dust mites there was a significant difference between treatment and control groups (−0.50, −0.98 to −0.01) which favoured the control group (one of the two studies had a baseline difference which favoured the control group[9]). In the analysis of five crossover trials of physical methods the difference was 0.06 (−0.26 to 0.37) (fig 3); for the only parallel group trial the difference was 0.33 (−0.28 to

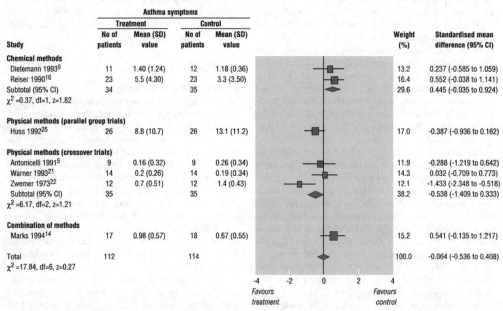

Fig 2 Standardised mean difference (95% confidence interval) in asthma symptoms after the use of either chemical or physical methods to reduce exposure to house dust mites. Negative values indicate that treatment is better than control

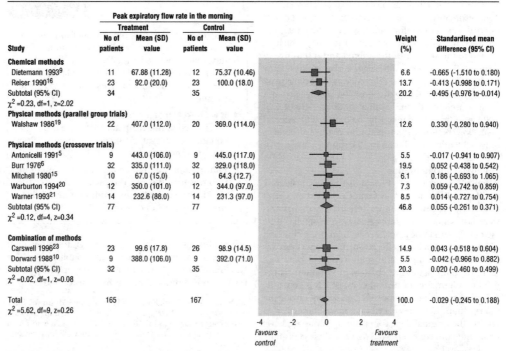

	Peak expiratory flow rate in the morning						
	Treatment		Control			Weight	Standardised mean
Study	No of patients	Mean (SD) value	No of patients	Mean (SD) value		(%)	difference (95% CI)
Chemical methods							
Dietemann 1993[9]	11	67.88 (11.28)	12	75.37 (10.46)		6.6	-0.665 (-1.510 to 0.180)
Reiser 1990[16]	23	92.0 (20.0)	23	100.0 (18.0)		13.7	-0.413 (-0.998 to 0.171)
Subtotal (95% CI)	34		35			20.2	-0.495 (-0.976 to -0.014)
χ^2 =0.23, df=1, z=2.02							
Physical methods (parallel group trials)							
Walshaw 1986[19]	22	407.0 (112.0)	20	369.0 (114.0)		12.6	0.330 (-0.280 to 0.940)
Physical methods (crossover trials)							
Antonicelli 1991[5]	9	443.0 (106.0)	9	445.0 (117.0)		5.5	-0.017 (-0.941 to 0.907)
Burr 1976[6]	32	335.0 (111.0)	32	329.0 (118.0)		19.5	0.052 (-0.438 to 0.542)
Mitchell 1980[15]	10	67.0 (15.0)	10	64.3 (12.7)		6.1	0.186 (-0.693 to 1.065)
Warburton 1994[20]	12	350.0 (101.0)	12	344.0 (97.0)		7.3	0.059 (-0.742 to 0.859)
Warner 1993[21]	14	232.6 (88.0)	14	231.3 (97.0)		8.5	0.014 (-0.727 to 0.754)
Subtotal (95% CI)	77		77			46.8	0.055 (-0.261 to 0.371)
χ^2 =0.12, df=4, z=0.34							
Combination of methods							
Carswell 1996[23]	23	99.6 (17.8)	26	98.9 (14.5)		14.9	0.043 (-0.518 to 0.604)
Dorward 1988[10]	9	388.0 (106.0)	9	392.0 (71.0)		5.5	-0.042 (-0.966 to 0.882)
Subtotal (95% CI)	32		35			20.3	0.020 (-0.460 to 0.499)
χ^2 =0.02, df=1, z=0.08							
Total	165		167			100.0	-0.029 (-0.245 to 0.188)
χ^2 =5.62, df=9, z=0.26							

-4   -2   0   2   4
Favours control   Favours treatment

Fig 3 Standardised mean difference (95% confidence interval) of peak expiratory flow rate in the morning after the use of either chemical or physical methods to reduce exposure to house dust mites. Positive values indicate that treatment is better than control

0.94).[19] For the two studies evaluating a combination of methods the difference was 0.02 (−0.46 to 0.50).

Peak expiratory flow in the evening was only reported in six trials[5 9 10 15 20 21]; the difference was −0.13 (−0.48 to 0.22). For the only study that reported on chemical methods the difference was −1.08 (−1.97 to −0.20) in favour of the control group.[9] For physical methods of control the difference was 0.06 (−0.35 to 0.47). For the trials evaluating a combination of methods it was −0.03 (−0.96 to 0.89). The difference for forced expiratory volume in 1 second was 0.09 (−0.16 to 0.33).

There was no difference between the treatments in their effects on provocative concentration (standardised mean difference 0.04, −0.32 to 0.23) or use of drugs (−0.14, −0.43 to 0.15). Data for chemical methods were given only in one study in which the use of anti-asthma drugs was significantly higher in the treatment group (0.89, 0.02 to 1.75).[9]

None of the studies reported on the number of unscheduled visits made to a doctor or hospital. One study reported that three patients missed school during the control period and none missed school during treatment but did not give reasons for these differences.[22] Results of skin prick testing after treatment were not reported in any study.

In the subgroup of trials that reported a successful reduction in the population of mites the results were similar to the overall results.[10 11 19 21 23 25] For measures of morning peak flow rate the difference was 0.11 (−0.22 to 0.45). The only parallel group trial in this subgroup had a baseline difference that favoured the experimental group[19]; if this trial is excluded the difference becomes 0.02 (−0.39 to 0.42).

Discussion

We were unable to show any clinical benefit from measures designed to reduce exposure to mites among asthma patients who were sensitive to mites. Since patients with asthma are frequently sensitive to house dust mite allergen, the most likely explanation for our negative findings is that the methods studied did not adequately reduce levels of mite antigens. Those few studies in which exposure to mites was effectively reduced did not have results that were more positive than studies in which exposure to mites was not reduced. This may be because patients with asthma who are sensitive to mites are usually also sensitive to other allergens; the successful elimination of only one allergen may be of limited benefit.

It seems unlikely that the initial levels of mite infestation were already too low for any reduction to be effective. Quite low concentrations of allergen can affect bronchial responsiveness,[27 28] and the concentrations in the studies reviewed would usually represent a risk to patients sensitive to mites.

A lack of compliance with the measures to control mites could have played a part in the negative results, but only in one study[25] was adherence to protocols evaluated. Adherence to protocols was higher and the amount of mites patients were exposed to was lower in the group that received computer assisted instruction when compared with the group that received conventional instruction. Those subjects who received computer assisted instruction implemented significantly more avoidance measures and had fewer symptoms.

Our meta-analysis did not seem to lack power. The point estimates were close to zero and the confidence interval was narrow for morning peak flow rate, the most commonly used outcome measure, which is related to the severity of the asthma and is sensitive to change. This does not suggest we missed any worthwhile effect. If the difference in morning peak flow is transformed into the most commonly used unit of measurement (l/min) with a standard deviation of 100 l/min (in accordance with fig 3), the difference in peak flow between treatment and control groups is only -3 l/min (-25 l/min to 19 l/min).

Potential sources of bias

Potential sources of bias must be considered. Randomisation methods were not reported except in one study. In several studies researchers or patients were not blinded, and most studies were small. These factors all tend to be associated with an overestimation of reported treatment effects. Further, reporting was variable (for example, one study reported only that there were no significant changes in symptom scores, drug requirements, or peak flow rates[13]). It is generally safe to assume that unreported data do not favour the intervention. On a few occasions it was necessary to correct the original data; for example, in one study we could not confirm a reported significant effect on mite allergen level.[12]

We tried to avoid bias while extracting data (for example, by making blinded decisions when several options were available). On a few occasions, however, we had to use data that favoured the experimental interventions (appendix 1 on the website). Finally, the trials we excluded did not have positive results (appendix 2 on the website) and we therefore believe we have not favoured the null hypothesis of no treatment effect in our meta-analysis.

There is a possibility that the results of effective interventions have been diluted by ineffective ones or by trial designs that were insufficiently rigorous. The length of follow up varied but was completely unrelated to the effect of treatment (for example, the three trials with 6-12 months of follow up showed a difference of 0.01 (-0.36 to 0.38) in morning peak flow). This is to be expected since an effect on the reduction of allergens should be noticeable in the short term because mite allergen causes a Type I hypersensitivity reaction. There may be a subset of patients who are highly sensitive to mites who would benefit from mite eradication. It would, however, be difficult to detect such patients and it seems more reasonable to assess the effects of mite eradication on all patients with asthma whose skin prick tests indicate a sensitivity to mites.

Conclusion

Current chemical and physical methods for eradicating mites or reducing exposure to mites seem to be ineffective and cannot be recommended as prophylactic treatment for asthma patients who are sensitive to mites. It is doubtful whether conducting further studies similar to the ones in our meta-analysis would be worthwhile. In particular, several of the trials had used extensive mite eradication and avoidance schemes. We suggest that future studies should be much larger and more rigorous than those analysed here and should

---

Key messages

- Current chemical and physical methods aimed at reducing exposure to allergens from house dust mites seem to be ineffective; these methods cannot be recommended as prophylactic treatment for asthma patients who are sensitive to mites

- It is unlikely that a worthwhile effect has been overlooked in this meta-analysis since the confidence interval for the peak expiratory flow rate was quite narrow

- Future studies should be much larger and more rigorous than those in this meta-analysis and should evaluate other methods of mite control than those used to date

---

use methods to control or eradicate mites other than those used so far. Our review is also published in The Cochrane Library[29] where it will be updated when results from additional studies become available.

We would like to thank Professor Paul W Jones, Mr Steve Milan, Ms Anna Bara, and Dr Jane Dennis, of the Cochrane Airways Group; Professor Vinod K Diwan and Professor Martin Bland for helpful support; and Dr Leonardo Antonicelli for providing additional data.

Contributors: CH wrote the draft protocol for the meta-analysis. CH and MB selected trials for inclusion. Trials were reviewed by all authors. Quality assessment of the trials was primarily done by CH, outcome data were extracted primarily by PCG (but discussed in detail with all authors), CH drafted the first manuscript for the Cochrane Library, PCG drafted the manuscript for the journal article. All authors are guarantors for the article, and PCG is guarantor for the statistical calculations.

Funding: Nordic Council of Ministers; Hovedstadens Sygehusfaellesskab, Rigshospitalet, Denmark; Sygekassernes Helsefond, Denmark; the Swedish Heart Lung Foundation (grant 54506).

Conflict of interest: None.

1 Custovic A, Simpson A, Chapman MD, Woodcock A. Allergen avoidance in the treatment of asthma and atopic disorders. *Thorax* 1998;53:63-72.
2 *Review manager: version 3.1 for Windows.* Oxford: Cochrane Collaboration, 1998. (Available from: www.cochrane.dk.)
3 Bland JM, Altman DG. Measurement error proportional to the mean. *BMJ* 1996;313:106.
4 Gøtzsche PC. Bias in double-blind trials. *Dan Med Bull* 1990;37:329-36.
5 Antonicelli L, Bilo MB, Pucci S, Schou C, Bonifazi F. Efficacy of an air-cleaning device equipped with a high efficiency particulate air filter in house dust mite respiratory allergy. *Allergy* 1991;46:594-600.
6 Burr ML, St Leger AS, Neale E. Anti-mite measurements in mite-sensitive adult asthma: a controlled trial. *Lancet* 1976;1:333-5.
7 Burr ML, Dean BV, Merrett TG, Neale E, St Leger AS, Verrier-Jones ER. Effects of anti-mite measures on children with mite-sensitive asthma: a controlled trial. *Thorax* 1980;35:506-12.
8 Burr ML, Neale E, Dean BV, Verrier-Jones ER. Effect of a change to mite-free bedding on children with mite-sensitive asthma: a controlled trial. *Thorax* 1980;35:513-4.
9 Dietemann A, Bessot JC, Hoyet C, Ott M, Verot A, Pauli G. A double-blind, placebo controlled trial of solidified benzyl benzoate applied in dwellings of asthmatic patients sensitive to mites: clinical efficacy and effect on mite allergens. *J Allergy Clin Immunol* 1993;91:738-46.
10 Dorward AJ, Colloff MJ, MacKay NS, McSharry C, Thomson NC. Effect of house dust mite avoidance measures on adult atopic asthma. *Thorax* 1988;43:98-102.
11 Ehnert B, Lau-Schadendorf S, Weber A, Buettner P, Schou C, Wahn U. Reducing domestic exposure to dust mite allergen reduces bronchial hyperreactivity in sensitive children with asthma. *J Allergy Clin Immunol* 1992;90:135-8.
12 Geller-Bernstein C, Pibourdin JM, Dornelas A, Fondarai J. Efficacy of the acaricide: Acardust for the prevention of asthma and rhinitis due to dust mite allergy in children. *Allergie et Immunologie* 1995;27:147-54.
13 Gillies DRN, Littlewood JM, Sarsfield JK. Controlled trial of house dust mite avoidance in children with mild to moderate asthma. *Clin Allergy* 1987;17:105-11.
14 Marks GB, Tovey ER, Green W, Shearer M, Salome CM, Woolcock AJ. House dust mite allergen avoidance: a randomised controlled trial of surface chemical treatment and encasement of bedding. *Clin Exp Allergy* 1994;24:1078-83.

15 Mitchell EA, Elliott RB. Controlled trial of an electrostatic precipitator in childhood asthma. *Lancet* 1980;2:559-61.
16 Reiser J, Ingram D, Mitchell EB, Warner JO. House dust mite allergen levels and an anti-mite mattress spray (natamycin) in the treatment of childhood asthma. *Clin Exp Allergy* 1990;20:561-7.
17 Sette L, Comis A, Marcucci F, Sensi L, Piacentini GL, Boner AL. Benzylbenzoate foam: effects on mite allergens in mattress, serum and nasal secretory IgE to Dermatophagoides pteronyssinus, and bronchial hyperreactivity in children with allergic asthma. *Pediatr Pulmonol* 1994;18:218-27.
18 Verrall B, Muir DCF, Wilson WM, Milner R, Johnston M, Dolovitch J. Laminar flow air cleaner bed attachment: a controlled trial. *Ann Allergy* 1988;61:117-22.
19 Walshaw MJ, Evans CC. Allergen avoidance in house dust mite sensitive adult asthma. *Q J Med* 1986;58:199-215.
20 Warburton CJ, Niven RMcL, Pickering CAC, Fletcher AM, Hepworth J, Francis HC. Domiciliary air filtration units, symptoms and lung function in atopic asthmatics. *Respir Med* 1994;88:771-6.
21 Warner JA, Marchant JL, Warner JO. Double blind trial of ionisers in children with asthma sensitive to the house dust mite. *Thorax* 1993;48:330-3.
22 Zwemer RJ, Karibo J. Use of laminar control device as adjunct to standard environmental control measures in symptomatic asthmatic children. *Ann Allergy* 1973;31:284-90.
23 Carswell F, Birmingham K, Oliver J, Crewes A, Weeks J. The respiratory

effects of reduction of mite allergen in the bedrooms of asthmatic children: a double-blind controlled trial. *Clin Exp Allergy* 1996;26:386-96.
24 Van der Heide S, Kaufmann HF, Dubois AEJ, de Monchy JGR. Allergen-avoidance measures in homes of house-dust-mite-allergic asthmatic patients: effects of acaricides and mattress encasings. *Allergy* 1997;52:921-7.
25 Huss K, Squire EN, Carpenter GB, Smith LJ, Huss RW, Salata K, et al. Effective education of adults with asthma who are allergic to dust mites. *J Allergy Clin Immunol* 1992;89:836-43.
26 Maesen FPV, Sluysmans FG, Brombacher PJ, Smeets JJ. Ervaringen met het gebruik van luchtfiltratieapparatuur in de woonruimten van voor huisstof overgevoelige atopische patienten. *Acta Tuberc Pneumol Belg* 1977;68:133-47.
27 Ihre E, Axelsson IGK, Zetterström O. Late asthmatic reactions and bronchial variability after challenge with low doses of allergen. *Clin Allergy* 1988;18:557-67.
28 Ihre E, Zetterstrom O. Increase in non-specific bronchial responsiveness after repeated inhalation of low doses of allergen. *Clin Exp Allergy* 1993;23:298-305.
29 Hammarquist C, Burr ML, Gøtzsche PC. House dust mite control measures in the management of asthma. In: *The Cochrane Library*, Issue 3. Oxford: Update Software, 1998.

(Accepted 28 July 1998)

Science commentary: Hypersensitivity revisited

When someone who is allergic to house dust mites starts wheezing they are experiencing a type I hypersensitivity reaction. Type I reactions occur rapidly and are mediated by IgE antibodies (to the allergen) which bind strongly to the surface of mast cells in the skin. The synthesis of IgE antibodies is triggered by T helper cells (Th 2 cells) which produce a number of inflammatory cytokines in the process. The most important cytokine in these type I responses is interleukin 4.

When the IgE antibodies bind to mast cells they break open and release histamine which causes the clinical symptoms. The clinical response usually stops when the allergen is removed or when the inflammatory response is dampened down by antihistamine drugs or anti-inflammatory drugs. Other type I hyper-

sensitivity reactions include allergic rhinitis, eczema, urticaria, and systemic anaphylaxis.

Type II and type III hypersensitivity reactions are mediated by IgG antibodies. These set off the complement cascade which induces phagocytosis of the allergens. Common examples of these hypersensitivity reactions include reactions to drugs and serum sickness. Type II reactions are directed against antigens on the cell surface; type III reactions are directed against soluble antigens.

Type IV hypersensitivity reactions are mediated by T cells, and tissue damage is caused by macrophages and cytotoxic T cells. Contact dermatitis is a clinical example of a type IV hypersensitivity reaction.

Abi Berger *Science editor, BMJ*

Meta-analysis: Unresolved issues and future developments

George Davey Smith, *professor of clinical epidemiology,*[a] **Matthias Egger**, *reader in social medicine and epidemiology* [a]

[a] Department of Social Medicine, University of Bristol, Bristol BS8 2PR
Correspondence to: Professor Davey Smith zetkin@bristol.ac.uk

Introduction

Since its recent introduction into clinical epidemiology, meta-analysis has established itself as an influential branch of biostatistics. Several books have focused mainly or entirely on meta-analysis in medicine,[1 2 3 4 5] and the latest editions of relevant textbooks generally include a section on meta-analysis. [6 7 8 9] Computer software entirely devoted to meta-analysis has been developed, and meta-analytic procedures have been introduced in general statistical software packages. We will soon be providing an overview of software packages on the *BMJ*'s website.[10] Several unresolved issues concerning meta-analysis remain, and in this final article of our series we address some of the topics that are likely to feature in future discussions of the appropriate practice and domain of meta-analysis.

Should unpublished data be included in meta-analyses?

Publication bias, discussed in detail in a previous article,[11] is a major threat to the validity of meta-analysis. Obtaining and including data from unpublished studies seems to be the obvious way of avoiding this problem. Including data from unpublished studies can itself introduce bias, however. Even after extensive consultation with the research community, unpublished studies may remain hidden. The unpublished studies that can be located may thus be an unrepresentative sample of unpublished studies. Whether bias is reduced or increased by including unpublished studies cannot formally be assessed as it is impossible to be certain that all unpublished studies have been located. A further problem relates to the willingness of investigators of located unpublished studies to provide data. This may depend on the findings of the study, more favourable results being provided more readily. This could again bias the findings of a meta-analysis.

Originally published in *BMJ* 1998; **316**: 760–2.

Summary points

Meta-analysis has established itself as an important technique in clinical epidemiology, but several issues remain unresolved

The inclusion of unpublished, non-peer reviewed data can be problematic, particularly if these data come from interested sources, such as the pharmaceutical industry

Individual patient data are often required to address important questions, but the mechanisms to facilitate increasing availability of trial data for meta-analysis are lacking

The clinical application of results from meta-analyses to the individual patient often remains a difficult matter of judgment

The Cochrane Collaboration will have an important role in future developments in the field of systematic reviews and meta-analyses

An analysis of 150 meta-analyses published between 1988 and 1991 showed that most meta-analysts had searched for unpublished material, although such data were located and included in only 31% of meta-analyses.[12] A questionnaire assessing the attitudes towards inclusion of unpublished data was sent to the authors of these reports and to the editors of the journals that had published them: 78% of meta-analysts supported the use of unpublished material, compared with only 47% of journal editors.[12] This lack of support by some editors is on the grounds that the data have not been peer reviewed. The refereeing process, however, has not always been a successful way of ensuring that published results are valid.[13][14] On the other hand, meta-analyses of unpublished data from interested sources is clearly of concern. Such unchallengeable data have been produced in circumstances in which an obvious commercial interest exists (box 1 gives an example).

Box 1: Controversy over selective serotonin uptake inhibitors and depression

- Selective serotonin uptake inhibitors are widely used for the treatment of depression, although their clinical advantages over the much less expensive tricyclic antidepressants have not been well established.

- In their meta-analysis Song et al used the dropout rate among randomised controlled trial participants taking selective serotonin uptake inhibitors and those taking conventional antidepressants as an indicator of therapeutic success[15]: patients who stop taking their treatment because of inefficacy or side effects are the ones who are not benefiting, and thus the class of drug with the lower dropout rate can be considered the one with the more favourable effects.

- There was little difference between selective serotonin uptake inhibitors and the other—usually tricyclic—antidepressants. In response to this analysis, Nakielny (for Lilly Industries, the manufacturers of fluoxetine) presented a meta-analysis of 14 investigational studies of new drugs which they stated included every study completed by December 1990.[16] This included what were called "unpublished data on file." The pooled dropout rates calculated by Nakielny differed markedly from the literature based analysis.

121

| | No of trials | Fluoxetine | | Tricyclic antidepressant | | |
		No of patients	Drop out rate (%)	No of patients	Drop out rate (%)	P value
Song et al [15]	18*	913	34.5	916	36.7	0.4
Nakielny[16]	14	781	36.5	788	47.5	<0.0001

*References 6, 12-15, 18, 29, 31, 33-35, 44, 47, 63, 65-67, 69 in Song et al.[15]

Lilly Industries claimed that its analysis was not "subject to biases introduced by selective publication and literature searches," but this is difficult to assess if the trials included represent unpublished data "on file". To make such data available in the future is one of the major challenges facing meta-analysts and the promoters of systematic reviews and evidence based medicine.

The most satisfactory approach to the inclusion of unpublished data in meta-analyses is to carry out an extensive search for such data and obtain them if possible. The analysis should then be performed with and without the unpublished data, as a form of sensitivity analysis. If the conclusions are altered through the inclusion or exclusion of such data, the results of either approach should be treated cautiously.

▶ Subjectivity in data analysis and reporting

Using published results exclusively can introduce biases other than those of publication bias. The choice of the outcome that is reported can be influenced by the results: the outcome with the most favourable findings will generally be reported. An example of how published results can be misleading comes from two separate analyses of a double blind, placebo controlled trial assessing the efficacy of amoxycillin in children with non-suppurative otitis media.[17][18] Opposite conclusions were reached, mainly because different weight was given to the various outcome measures assessed in the study. This disagreement was conducted in the public arena, as it was accompanied by accusations of impropriety against the team producing the findings favourable to amoxycillin. The leader of this team had received considerable funding, both in research grants and as personal honorarium, from the manufacturers of amoxycillin.[19] This is a good example of how reliance on the data chosen to be presented by the investigators can lead to distortion.[20] This has probably been a frequent source of bias, which only in rare occasions becomes common knowledge. With improving standards of clinical trial reporting[21] subjectivity in data analysis shouldbecome less common in the future.

▶ Individual patient data or summary statistics—which should be included in a meta-analysis?

Meta-analyses that have been entirely dependent on summary data obtained from published reports of clinical trials have provided robust indicators of treatment outcomes. Such analyses have been described as meta-analyses of the literature.[22] If a researcher is interested in outcomes in different groups, however, the analysis will be made difficult if the various trials do not report data accordingly. For example, a literature based meta-analysis of the effect of drug treatment of hypertension in elderly people [23]was obliged to use a definition of "elderly" that included the participants aged 60 or over from some studies and those aged 65 or over from others. Also, because many trials failed to report age stratified data, less than half of the potential trials could be included in the analysis. This could create serious bias, as the decision of investigators to publish age stratified data may have been dependent on results.

Supplementary data from individual trials are increasingly being obtained for meta-analyses. For example, by obtaining data on mortality from coronary heart disease according to grouped follow up periods from the original investigators of cholesterol lowering trials, Law et al were able to show that the reduction in risk of coronary heart disease consequent on cholesterol lowering increased with the duration of treatment.[23] Several collaborative groups have assembled data on each participant within the separate trials. This greatly increases flexibility when defining groups within the different trials for subgroup analyses, and also allows use of data on the exact time to the event for each participant. For example, the Fibrinolytic Therapy Trialists' Collaborative Group investigated the effect of thrombolysis after myocardial infarction according to *(a)* the electrocardiographic abnormalities of patients at entry to the study; *(b)* the time at which treatment was received after onset of symptoms; *(c)* the age and sex of the patients; and *(d)* the presence or absence of various comorbid conditions.[24] This permits comparisons that retain the advantage of the original randomisation to be made, with the proviso that the separate trials did not necessarily use stratified randomisation according to these characteristics. Box 2 presents a further example.

Box 2: Coronary artery bypass graft surgery and survival: meta-analysis using individual patient data

- It has long been accepted that coronary artery bypass graft surgery provides effective relief from angina pectoris and that it prolongs survival in high risk patients with left main artery disease

- The effect of such surgery on survival in other categories of patients with coronary heart disease, however, remains controversial

- A meta-analysis of trials compared coronary artery bypass graft surgery with conventional treatment in patients with stable coronary heart disease.[25] The graft surgery overall was associated with a significant reduction of mortality—for example, at five years 10.2% *v* 15.8%, P=0.0001)

- For this meta-analysis the individual patient data made it possible to perform several subgroup analyses. For example, by using a modification of the veterans administration risk score[26] (which is based on the presence of class III or IV angina, ST depression at rest, history of hypertension, and history of myocardial infarction) the relation of benefit with the level of risk could be explored. No benefit was evident in the third at lowest risk, which was characterised by a relatively low five year mortality of 5.5%. Conversely, benefit was present for groups of patients at higher risk of death (1). This information is crucial to the clinical application of the results from meta-analyses, indicating that targeting coronary artery bypass graft surgery at high risk individuals would be an efficient way of using limited resources

- This example illustrates how important information can be derived from risk stratification based on individual patient data

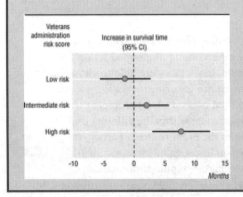

Obtaining individual patient data has advantages beyond the ability to perform standardised subgroup analyses.[27] Contact with individual investigators can help to identify further trials—published and unpublished—which the meta-analysts had missed. It may be possible to identify deviations from protocols in the trials—for example, participants who were included even though they did not satisfy entry criteria. Incorrect analyses—for example, deviation from "intention to treat" analysis, the presence of unreported dropouts, and simple oversights—may be identified. Outcome measures can be better standardised across the trials, which will counteract the tendency of researchers to publish the results only in terms of the most striking effect on a particular outcome. Additional follow up data can also be obtained, as for some trials the period of randomised comparison continues beyond the initial publication, but only the published data are publicly available.

Value of "failed" meta-analyses

In some cases a conclusive meta-analysis may not be possible if methodological standards are to be maintained. In such "failed" meta analyses[28] the treatment methods, concurrent treatment, length of follow up, characteristics of the study participants, or end points that were measured might be too varied to allow for the sensible combination of results. A meta-analysis exclusively based on a small number of trials will often have to be inconclusive, even if the combined estimate of effect is significant.[11 29]

The *Cochrane Database of Systematic Reviews* contains many examples of treatment interventions for which, the reviewers thought, meta-analysis had failed to produce a conclusive answer. For example, the review on thrombolysis in acute ischaemic stroke, published in the second issue of the

Cochrane Library in 1996,[30] stated: "...the data so far are scant, and quite insufficient to make any definite conclusion about the benefit or otherwise of thrombolysis to treat acute ischaemic stroke." Additional trials have since been published, and an updated version of the same review (issue 2, 1997) concluded that, although more research was needed, clear evidence existed for a substantial excess risk of intracranial haemorrhage and early death with high doses of thrombolytic drugs. Clearly stating and showing the inadequacy of existing evidence should serve as a stimulus for conducting the appropriate and necessary trials.

▶ The Cochrane Collaboration

The dissemination of failed reviews is an important task, which is neglected by traditional journals. The examples mentioned above illustrate that this is increasingly being taken on by the Cochrane Collaboration, along with the dissemination of many other, conclusive reviews. This international group, named after Archie Cochrane, is a unique initiative in the evaluation of healthcare interventions. In his seminal book *Effectiveness and Efficiency: Random Reflections on Health Services*, published in 1972, Cochrane forcefully argued that the healthcare resources should be used to provide equitably those interventions that have been shown in well designed studies to be effective.[31] The collaboration's effort to prepare, disseminate, and continuously update systematic reviews of controlled trials is an essential, and timely, step towards achieving this goal. The Cochrane Collaboration will have an important role in future developments in the field of systematic reviews and meta-analysis. The collaboration's working groups are addressing many of the currently unresolved issues, including, for example, the approach to observational data and data from evaluations of screening and diagnostic tests. Ways of improving the applicability of reviews, discussed below, and of strengthening the involvement of consumer representatives, are also being studied.

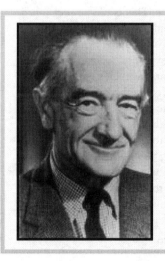

Archie Cochrane (1909–88), the pioneer in health services research whose visions are at the heart of the Cochrane Collaboration

▶ Clinical application of results from meta-analyses

Single large trials showing beneficial effects of treatments do influence medical practice, whereas meta-analyses of smaller studies have generally had limited impact. For example, the use of thrombolysis to reduce mortality from myocardial infarction increased only after publication of two large trials in the late 1980s,[32][33] although the same reduction in mortality had already been shown in 1982 in a meta-analysis of eight smaller studies[34] and again in a 1985 meta-analysis.[35] The increase in the use of thrombolysis is in line with the recommendations made in authoritative reviews and textbooks. Only after publication of the first trial by the Gruppo Italiano per lo Studio della Streptochinasi nell'Infarto Miocardico was thrombolysis increasingly recommended as routine treatment after myocardial infarction.[36] The 1982 meta-analysis has received only 150 citations over the 14 years since its publication in the *New England Journal of Medicine* (the medical journal with the highest impact factor), whereas the 1985 meta-analysis has received about 350 citations, the same as those received by a small, inconclusive trial that was published in the same year.[37] The two large trials, however, have received several thousand citations over a shorter period. Clearly, meta-analyses, even when conclusive, currently receive less attention than the trials which they pool, and this is presumably reflected in a smaller degree of influence on clinical practice.

Clinicians want results from clinical research that can usefully inform their clinical practice. Perhaps meta-analyses are seen as not providing information beyond the effect of treatment on a hypothetical "average" patient. The confidence interval, often narrow in meta-analysis, reflects how certain one can be about the size of the overall effect seen in a population. Of more relevance to the clinician, however, is how certain one can be about the effect in his or her particular patient. Although the overall effect will generally provide the best available estimate, the uncertainty with respect to a particular patient will always be greater than with respect to the overall patient group. This is because, in the same way as the effect under examination varies between the component studies in the meta-analysis, the effect further varies between different patients.[38]

Many clinical opinion leaders simply do not trust the results from meta-analyses. This could be seen as a cautious attitude to a relatively new technique, which is justified considering the existence of misleading meta-analyses.[29][39] The emergence of the "professional meta-analyst"[40] moving monthly from issue to issue, happily engaging in areas outside their domain of primary expertise, filling the pages of the medical journals, and sometimes viewed as lackeys for governmental agencies with a cost cutting agenda, has certainly not helped here. We believe that with improved methodological standards that routinely involve thorough sensitivity analyses, confidence in the results from meta-analyses will gradually grow. Although knowledge of the accumulated evidence from clinical trials should certainly provide a strong guide for practice, it is appropriate that features of the particular clinical situation should also be incorporated into the decision making process. The failure to recognise that the world is characterised as much by difference as similarity, which may be lost to those faced by numbers not patients, has on occasion led to overconfident assertions from practitioners of meta-analysis, which have understandably antagonised clinicians. Retaining a degree of humility in the face of the diversity of humanity served by medicine, and thus admitting to greater uncertainty than may be wished, will in the end prove the best way of furthering the goals of meta-analysis and the practice of evidence-based medicine to which it contributes.

▶ Outlook

In this series we outlined and illustrated the principles, strengths, and weaknesses of meta-analysis. We believe that this technique is clearly superior to the narrative approach to reviewing medical research. In addition to providing a precise estimate of the overall treatment effect in some instances, appropriate examination of heterogeneity across individual studies can produce clinically useful information with which to guide rational and cost effective treatment decisions. Both the uncritical synthesis of data from observational studies and the unconsidered synthesis of disparate results from randomised controlled trials threaten to damage the reputation of meta-analysis.

Some of the shortcomings of meta-analysis, however, are a consequence of a more general failing with respect to the dissemination of research findings. Currently this process is highly dependent on the publication of study results in peer reviewed, English-language journals. Considerations regarding publication and location biases have shown that this can result in a selected portion of all the evidence becoming available for systematic review. This is clearly unsatisfactory and can misdirect clinical practice, whether or not a formal meta-analysis is performed. Meta-analyses based on individual patient data have shown that making such data available can contribute valuable and clinically relevant information that could not be obtained from published sources. Mechanisms to facilitate such collaborative analyses and to ensure wide accessibility of results from clinical research, including results kept as "data on file" by the pharmaceutical industry, must be developed further. The technological barriers to worldwide data exchange and collaboration are tumbling down—we can only hope that the remaining barriers, rooted in customary practice, political agendas, and commercial interests, will swiftly fall too.

▶ Acknowledgements

The department of social medicine at the University of Bristol is part of the Medical Research Council's health services research collaboration.

▶ References

1. Petitti DB. *Meta-analysis, decision analysis, and cost-effectiveness analysis. Methods for quantitative synthesis in medicine.* New York: Oxford University Press, 1994.
2. Warren KS, Mosteller F, eds. *Doing more good than harm. The evaluation of health care interventions.* New York: New York Academy of Sciences, 1993.
3. Cooper H, Hedges LV, eds. *The handbook of research synthesis.* New York: Russell Sage Foundation, 1994.
4. Hedges LV, Olkin I. *Statistical methods for meta-analysis.* Boston: Academic Press, 1985.
5. Eddy DM, Hasselblad V, Shachter R. *Meta-analysis by the confidence profile method. The statistical synthesis of evidence.* Boston: Academic Press, 1992.
6. Armitage P, Berry G. *Statistical methods in medical research.* Oxford: Blackwell Science, 1994.
7. Altman DG. *Practical statistics for medical research.* London: Chapman and Hall, 1991.
8. Lilienfeld DE, Stolley PD. *Foundations of epidemiology.* New York: Oxford University Press, 1994.
9. Davey Smith G, Egger M, Phillips AN. Meta-analysis and data synthesis in medical research. In: Detels R, Holland WW, McEwen J, Omenn GS, eds. *Oxford textbook of public*

127

health . New York: Oxford University Press (in press).

10. Egger M, Davey Smith G. Meta-analysis software (http.www.bmj.com).

11. Egger M, Davey Smith G. Meta-analysis: bias in location and selection of studies. *BMJ* 1998;**316**:61–6.

12. Cook DJ, Guyatt GH, Ryan G, Clifton J, Buckingham L, Willan A, et al. Should unpublished data be included in meta-analyses? Current convictions and controversies. *JAMA* 1993;**269**:2749–53.

13. Rennie D. Problems in peer review and fraud: cleave ever to the sunnier side of doubt. In: *Balancing act. Essays to honour Stephen Lock.* London: Keynes Press, 1991.

14. Nylenna M, Riis P, Karlsson Y. Multiple blinded reviews of the same two manuscripts: effects of referee characteristics and publication language. *JAMA* 1994;**272**:149–51.

15. Song F, Freemantle N, Sheldon TA, House A, Watson P, Long A, et al. Selective serotonin reuptake inhibitors: meta-analysis of efficacy and acceptability. *BMJ* 1993;**306**:683–7.

16. Nakielny J. Effective and acceptable treatment for depression. *BMJ* 1993;**306**:1125.

17. Mandel EH, Rockette HE, Bluestone CD, Paradise JL, Nozza RJ. Efficacy of amoxicillin with and without decongestant-antihistamine for otitis media with effusion in children. *New Engl J Med* 1987;**316**:432–7.

18. Cantekin EI, McGuire TW, Griffith TL. Antimicrobial therapy for otitits media with effusion ("secretory" otitits media). *JAMA* 1991;**266**:3309–17.

19. Rennie D. The Cantekin affair. *JAMA* 1991;**266**:3333–7.

20. Subjectivity in data analysis [editorial]. *Lancet* 1991;**337**:401–2.

21. Begg CB, Cho M, Eastwood S, Horton R, Moher D, Olkin I, et al. Improving the quality of reporting of randomized controlled trials. The CONSORT statement. *JAMA* 1996;**276**:637–9.

22. Stewart LA, Parmar MKB. Meta-analysis of the literaure or of individual patient data: is there a difference? *Lancet* 1993;**341**:418–22.

25. Yusuf S, Zucker D, Peduzzi P, Fisher LD, Takaro T, Kennedy JW, et al. Effect of coronary artery bypass graft surgery on survival: overview of 10-year results from randomised trials by the Coronary Artery Graft Surgery Trialists Collaboration. *Lancet* 1994;**344**:563–70.

26. Takaro T, Hultgren HN, Lipton MJ, Detre KM. The VA cooperative randomized study of surgery for coronary arterial occlusive disease II: subgroup with significant left main lesions. *Circulation* 1976;**54**(suppl 3):107–17.

27. Clarke MJ, Stewart LA. Systematic reviews: obtaining data from randomised controlled trials: how much do we need for reliable and informative meta-analyses? *BMJ* 1994;**309**:1007–10.

28. Naylor CD. The case for failed meta-analyses. *J Clin Eval Clin Pract* 1995;1:127–30.

29. Egger M, Davey Smith G, Schneider M, Minder CE. Bias in meta-analysis detected by a simple, graphical test. *BMJ*;**315**:629–34.

30. Wardlaw J, Yamaguchi T, del Zoppo G, Hacke W. Thrombolysis in acute ischaemic stroke. In: Warlow C, van Gijn J, Sandercock P, eds. *Stroke Module of the Cochrane Database of Systematic Reviews, [updated 03 June 1996]. Available in The Cochrane Library [database on disk and CD ROM]. The Cochrane Collaboration; Issue 2.* Oxford: Update Software, 1996.

31. Cochrane A. *Effectiveness and efficiency. Random reflections on health services.* London: Nuffield Provincial Hospital Trust, 1972.

32. Gruppo Italiano per lo Studio della Streptochinasi nell'Infarto Miocardico (GISSI). Effectiveness of intravenous thrombolytic treatment in acute myocardial infarction. *Lancet* 1986;**397**–402.

33. ISIS-2 Collaborative Group. Randomised trial of intravenous streptokinase, oral aspirin, both, or neither among 17,187 cases of suspected acute myocardial infarction: ISIS-2. *Lancet* 1988;ii:349–60.

34. Stampfer MJ, Goldhaber SZ, Yusuf S, Peto R, Hennekens CH. Effect of intravenous streptokinase on acute myocardial infarction. Pooled results from randomized trials. *New Engl J Med* 1982;**307**:1180–2.

35. Yusuf S, Collins R, Peto R, Furberg C, Stampfer MJ, Goldhaber SZ, et al. Intravenous and intracoronary fibrinolytic therapy in acute myocardial infarction: overview of results on mortality, reinfarction and side-effects from 33 randomized controlled trials. *Eur Heart J* 1985;**6**:556–85.

36. Antman EM, Lau J, Kupelnick B, Mosteller F, Chalmers TC. A comparison of results of meta-analyses of randomized control trials and recommendations of clinical experts. *JAMA* 1992;**268**:240–8.
37. Simoons ML, Serruys PW, van den Brand M, Bar F, de Zwaan C, Res J, et al. Improved survival after early thrombolysis in acute myocardial infarction. *Lancet* 1985;ii:578–82.
38. Gelber RD, Goldhirsch A. From the overview to the patient: how to interpret meta-analysis data. *Recent Results in Cancer Research* 1993;**127**:167–76.
39. Egger M, Davey Smith G. Misleading meta-analysis. Lessons from "an effective, safe, simple" intervention that wasn't. *BMJ* 1995;**310**:752–4.
40. Rosendaal FR. The emergence of a new species: the professional meta-analyst. *J Clin Epidemiol* 1994;**47**:1325–6.

Papers that go beyond numbers (qualitative research)

BACKGROUND

Qualitative research is a "hot topic" in EBHC. "Evidence-based medicine" initially aligned itself with the sort of research evidence that could be expressed as mathematical estimates of risk and benefit in population samples. More recently, the value of qualitative research has been recognised for expanding our understanding of, for example, the experience of illness, the appropriateness of health services, and the barriers to change in patients and professionals. But just because qualitative research is becoming popular does not mean that all published qualitative studies are valid and relevant!

SUGGESTED AIM FOR THIS SESSION

For participants to develop, and feel confident in helping others to develop, the ability to determine whether the results and conclusions of a research article describing qualitative research are valid and applicable to their own practice and to address the implications of that study for further research.

SUGGESTED LEARNING OBJECTIVES FOR THIS SESSION

By the end of this session, participants should be able to evaluate a paper on qualitative research and in particular to:
- decide whether a qualitative, quantitative or combined approach should have been used for the problem being addressed;
- determine the perspective of the researcher(s) and decide how this is likely to have influenced the findings;
- decide whether the methods used were valid;
- decide whether the conclusions are justified;
- estimate the extent to which the findings are transferable to other settings;
- comment critically on the potential application and implementation of the results.

SET ARTICLES

Ruston A, Clayton J, Calnan M. Patients' action during their cardiac event: qualitative study exploring differences and modifiable factors. *BMJ* 1998; **316**: 1060–4.
Green J. Commentary: grounded theory and the constant group method. *BMJ* 1998; **316**: 1064–5.

ADDITIONAL REPRINT

Green J, Britten N. Qualitative research and evidence based medicine. *BMJ* 1998; **316**: 1230–2.

Clinical scenario

Bob Cookson, a 54-year-old bricklayer, develops severe central chest pain while at work. Since the pain came on while eating lunch, his two colleagues decide that "it must have been something he ate". Bob concurs with this, saying, "It can't be my heart – it's not on the left hand side". His friends sit with him for two hours until the pain begins to subside, then they allow him to go home unaccompanied on the bus. Unfortunately, he collapses with further pain soon afterwards and quickly loses consciousness. He is pronounced dead on arrival at hospital.

SUGGESTIONS FOR GROUP EXERCISES

When you have read the paper, try one or more of the following.
1. Use the paper in a training situation where a consultant in accident and emergency medicine is teaching a group of new registrars about patients' concerns (and lack of them) when they develop chest pain.
2. Have a debate or discussion (using role play if necessary to represent extreme positions) on the place of qualitative research in the "hierarchy of evidence".
3. Decide whether this paper should be used (a) to influence practice and policy directly, (b) to plan more "definitive" (quantitative) research into this issue or (c) neither.

SUGGESTIONS FOR INDIVIDUAL STUDY

Imagine you had written the set article yourself and submitted it to a hypothetical journal entitled *Important Scientific Findings in Cardiology*. The paper is rejected on the grounds that it is not a randomised controlled trial. Write a letter to the editor appealing against the decision.

CRITICAL APPRAISAL CHECKLIST FOR AN ARTICLE ON QUALITATIVE RESEARCH	
Note that the questions on the checklist are really looking for problems of bias, confounding, low power, and poor validity.	
A. Was a qualitative approach appropriate?	**Yes/No/Don't know**
1. Did the study ask how or why something was taking place (e.g. how people experience illness, health services or how or why patients and health professionals behave the way they do)?	
2. Was there a clearly formulated question (which may have been extended, refined or modified as the results accumulated)?	
B. Was the sampling strategy clearly defined and justified	
3. Was the method of sampling (for both the subjects and the setting) adequately described?	

4. Did the investigators study a representative range of individuals and settings relevant to their question?	
5. Were the characteristics of the subjects defined?	
C. Has the researcher critically examined their own role, potential bias and influence?	
6. Has the researcher taken their background and perspective into account in the analysis? • Is there a clear statement on the researcher's background and perspective and how this is likely to have influenced the results?	
D. What methods did the researcher use for collecting data?	
7. Have appropriate data sources been studied? • Did the author conduct a literature search?	
8. Were the methods used reliable and independently verifiable? • Audiotape, videotape, field notes? • Were observations taken in a range of circumstances (e.g. at different times)? • Was more than one method of data collection used (triangulation)?	
E. What methods did the researcher use to analyse the data, and what quality control measures were implemented?	
9. Did the authors use systematic methods to reduce their own biases influencing the results? • Did more than one researcher independently perform the analysis? • Were explicit methods used to resolve differences of interpretation? • Were explicit methods used to address negative or discrepant results?	
F. What are the results?	
10. What are the main findings of the research? • Are they coherent? • Do they address the research question?	
11. Are the results credible? • Are they consistent with the data? • Is it possible to determine the source of data presented (e.g. by numbering of extracts)? • Is most or all of the information collected available for independent assessment?	
12. Have alternative explanations for the results been explored and discounted?	
G. Were conclusions valid?	
13. What were the authors' conclusions? • Were they consistent with the data and results?	
H. To what extent are the findings of the study transferable to other clinical settings?	
14. Were the subjects in the study similar in important respects to my own patients?	
15. Is the context similar to my own practice?	

FURTHER READING

Donald A, Greenhalgh T. *A hands-on guide to evidence-based health care: practice and implementation.* Oxford: Blackwell Science, 1999.

Giacomini MK, Cook DJ. A user's guide to qualitative research in health care. Part I: Are the results of the study valid? *JAMA* 1999; in press.

Giacomini MK, Cook DJ. A user's guide to qualitative research in health care. Part II: What are the results and how do they help me care for my patients? *JAMA* 1999; in press.

Greenhalgh T. *How to read a paper: the basics of evidence based medicine.* London: BMJ Books, 1997. See in particular Chapter 11: Papers that go beyond numbers, pages 151–62.

Patients' action during their cardiac event: qualitative study exploring differences and modifiable factors

Annmarie Ruston, Julie Clayton, Michael Calnan

Editorial by Evans

Centre for Health Services Studies, George Allen Wing, University of Kent at Canterbury, Canterbury CT2 7NF

Annmarie Ruston, *research fellow*

Julie Clayton, *research associate*

Michael Calnan, *professor*

Correspondence to: Dr Ruston a.ruston@ukc.ac.uk

BMJ 1998;316:1060–5

Abstract

Objectives: To explore the circumstances and factors that explain variations in response to a cardiac event and to identify potentially modifiable factors.

Design: Qualitative analysis of semistructured, face to face interviews with patients admitted to two district hospitals for a cardiac event and with other people present at the time of the event. Patients were divided into three groups according to the length of delay between onset of symptoms and calling for medical help.

Subjects: 43 patients and 21 other people present at the time of the cardiac event. Patients were divided into three groups according to the length of time between onset of symptoms and seeking medical help: non-delayers (<4 h; $n=21$), delayers (4-12 h; $n=12$), and extended delayers (>12 h; $n=10$).

Main outcome measures: Decision making process, strategies for dealing with symptoms, and perception of risk and of heart attacks before the event according to delay in seeking help.

Results: The illness and help seeking behaviour of informants had several components, including warning, interpretation, preliminary action, re-evaluation, and final action stages. The length of each stage was variable and depended on the extent to which informants mobilised and integrated resources into a strategy to bring their symptoms under control. There were obvious differences in informants' knowledge of the symptoms that they associated with a heart attack before the event. Non-delayers described a wider range of symptoms before their heart attack and twice as many (13) considered themselves to be potentially at risk of a heart attack compared with the other two groups. For most informants the heart attack differed considerably from their concept of a heart attack.

Conclusion: The most critical factor influencing the time between onset of symptoms and calling for professional medical help is that patients and others recognise their symptoms as cardiac in origin. This study suggests that various points of intervention in the decision making process could assist symptom recognition and therefore faster access to effective treatment.

Introduction

A critical factor in preventing premature death or disability from a heart attack is ensuring that patients receive effective treatment to reduce damage to the heart muscle. Thrombolysis can reduce the size of the clot and hence the amount of muscle damage, but it must be given early for maximal benefit.[1][2] Thus patients or their associates need to recognise the symptoms and call for appropriate help immediately. We sought to explain variation in response to a cardiac event and to identify modifiable factors.

Subjects and methods

The study was conducted in two district general hospitals with coronary care units in one health authority. The subjects of the study were all admitted patients who had survived a cardiac event, which for this study was defined as a suspected or confirmed acute myocardial infarction. One patient who was too ill to be interviewed on the fifth day after the event was excluded. An integral part of the research design was interviewing, whenever possible, anyone else present at the time of the cardiac event. Subjects were recruited over five separate weeks in summer and winter months to ensure the required diversity of experience of a cardiac event and access to medical services. The original study design was intended to include associates of patients who died before arrival at hospital, but we could not obtain full ethical clearance for this.

Before the main study a pilot study was undertaken in one of the hospitals. During one week eight patients surviving a cardiac event and their associates (four relatives) were interviewed. They were not included in the main study.

Forty three patients were identified from coronary care units, accident and emergency departments, and medical and surgical wards, to ensure total coverage. Twenty one relatives and bystanders were also recruited.

Interviews

Patients were approached three to four days after admission to hospital and interviewed on the fifth day. The interviews lasted between 45 and 60 minutes. Patients were interviewed alone in the morning, and the other people were interviewed in the afternoon of the same day before they visited the patient. The

Originally published in *BMJ* 1998; **316**: 1060–64.

emphasis in the interviews was on enabling the informants to give spontaneous accounts of their decision making at the time of the cardiac event. However, after thorough piloting we decided to add some direct questions about informants' beliefs and knowledge of cardiac events. The themes explored in the interviews covered what experiences and actions led up to the cardiac event; when informants thought that the cardiac event had begun, what they thought the problem was and why it had occurred; whom they talked to and the effect of this interaction; when the decision to call for medical help was made and by whom; and who was called. The more direct areas of questioning were informants' conception of risk factors; which groups of people they associated with heart attacks; their knowledge of symptoms before the event; their concept of a heart attack; their knowledge of thrombolytic treatment; their family history; and personal details, including risk factors.

Data analysis

The interviews were tape recorded and transcribed verbatim. Before analysis informants were divided into three groups according to the length of time between the onset of symptoms and seeking medical help. The delays were less than 4 hours (non-delayers), between 4 and 12 hours (delayers), and more than 12 hours (extended delayers). The division was prompted by current evidence, which suggests that the earlier thrombolytic treatment is given the greater the reduction in deaths[1] and that for patients presenting after 12 hours benefit is limited.[2] Of the patients interviewed, 21 were non-delayers, 12 delayers, and 10 extended delayers. The division of informants into these groups provided a basis for illustrating the differences between those who seek help quickly and those who do not.

The data were analysed using the constant comparative method to cover identified and emerging themes.[3] A further analysis was undertaken by a second researcher AR, who listened to the tape recordings and examined the data to ensure that concepts, relations between variables, differences between groups, and the division of informants into the groups were confirmed or modified if necessary. There was agreement over which groups patients belonged to in all but three cases.

Results

Forty patients were diagnosed as having a confirmed acute myocardial infarction, and 9 of them had had a previous infarction (5 were non-delayers (24%), 2 delayers (17%), and 2 extended delayers (20%)) (table 1). Three quarters of the non-delayers were men (16/21) compared with 58% (7/12) of the delayers and 50% (5/10) of the extended delayers. A greater proportion of non-delayers were under 65 years of age compared with the other two groups (67% (14/21) v 58% (7/12) and 40% (4/10) respectively). A greater proportion of non-delayers also had manual occupations (62% (13/21) v 58% (7/12) and 50% (5/10) respectively).

Decision making process

The illness and help seeking behaviour of informants had several stages, including warning, interpretation,

Table 1 Characteristics of patients according to delay in seeking medical help for cardiac event

Case No	Age (years)	Sex	Acute myocardial infarction		Receiving treatment for CHD	Social group*
			Confirmed	Previous		
Non-delayers (<4 h)						
1	47	M	Yes	No	No	IV
2	65	F	Yes	Yes	Yes	V
3	79	F	Yes	No	No	V
4	55	M	Yes	No	No	IIIN
5	59	M	Yes	No	No	IIIN
6	52	M	Yes	No	No	II
7	64	M	Yes	No	No	IIIM
8	71	M	No	No	Yes	IV
9	50	M	Yes	No	No	IIIN
10	53	M	Yes	No	No	IIIM
11	75	M	Yes	Yes	Yes	IV
12	72	F	Yes	No	No	IV
13	52	F	Yes	No	No	IV
14	60	M	Yes	Yes	No	IV
15	59	M	Yes	Yes	Yes	IIIM
16	53	M	Yes	No	No	II
17	76	M	Yes	No	No	IIIN
18	64	M	Yes	No	No	IIIM
19	65	M	Yes	Yes	Yes	II
20	57	F	Yes	No	No	IV
21	60	M	Yes	No	No	IIIN
Delayers (4-12 h)						
22	53	F	No	No	No	IIIN
23	69	M	Yes	No	No	IV
24	74	F	Yes	No	No	IV
25	60	F	Yes	Yes	Yes	IV
26	71	F	Yes	No	Yes	IV
27	60	M	Yes	No	No	IIIN
28	49	M	Yes	No	No	IIIN
29	82	M	Yes	No	No	IIIM
30	48	M	Yes	No	No	II
31	55	M	Yes	No	No	IV
32	62	F	Yes	No	No	IV
33	80	M	Yes	Yes	Yes	II
Extended delayers (>12 h)						
34	71	F	Yes	No	No	IV
35	80	M	Yes	Yes	Yes	IIIM
36	73	M	No	No	Yes	IIIM
37	65	F	Yes	No	No	IIIN
38	56	M	Yes	No	No	IIIM
39	51	M	Yes	No	No	II
40	57	F	Yes	Yes	Yes	II
41	69	F	Yes	No	No	IV
42	75	F	Yes	No	Yes	II
43	63	M	Yes	No	No	II

CHD=coronary heart disease.
*Registrar general's classification.

preliminary action, re-evaluation, and final action. The length of each stage was variable and depended on the extent to which informants mobilised and integrated resources into a strategy to bring their symptoms under control. The time between onset of symptoms and calling for medical help was directly affected by the number and quality of the resources used in the individual strategy.

Five patients' symptoms were classically severe and unexpected and led them to respond quickly and call for medical help (cases 3, 4, 6, 20, and 21). The remaining patients experienced a warning stage in which symptoms were often intermittent and variable. The symptoms in many cases made the informants realise that they were not experiencing an episode from an

Table 2 Prevalence of symptoms during cardiac event according to delay in seeking medical help. Values are numbers (percentages) of patients

	Chest pain	Pain in neck and arms	Pain in arms	Sweating	Breathlessness	Nausea
Non-delayers (n=21)	20 (95)	6 (29)	6 (29)	10 (48)	6 (29)	2 (10)
Delayers (n=12)	11 (92)	8 (67)	8 (67)	5 (42)	6 (50)	2 (17)
Extended delayers (n=10)	9 (90)	3 (30)	8 (80)	5 (50)	7 (70)	3 (30)

acute illness but an evolving and cumulative event. During this stage patients treated themselves, referred to others, and in some cases sought medical help. For most patients, experience of symptoms before the acute phase had two effects: to increase tolerance of symptoms and to ensure that treatments were available to relieve symptoms during the acute event.

Table 2 shows the range of symptoms reported by informants. The range and severity of symptoms were similar in the three groups, symptoms initially being interpreted as common non-threatening problems by most informants. However, previous knowledge of the symptoms associated with a heart attack was noticeably different in the three groups. Non-delayers knew about a wide range of symptoms, including sweating, nausea, pains in the arms and neck, and breathing problems. Delayers generally knew only about chest and arm pain, while most extended delayers were unsure about symptoms.

Strategies for dealing with symptoms
Although most informants assigned an inappropriate diagnostic label to their symptoms at this stage, the strategy adopted for dealing with the symptoms delineated the three groups.

Non-delayers
The non-delayers generally entered a period of isolation and self evaluation, they did not consult with others, and only a few took any form of drug treatment. Most engaged in some form of diversion—for example, drinking cups of tea or moving about—while they evaluated the situation (box). In doing this, their symptoms were not masked and therefore escalated to a point where re-evaluation revealed the serious nature

---

Non-delayers: interpretation of symptoms

Taking stock
"I can't really explain how I felt, but I didn't feel well and I thought it was time to sit down and think about things. So, I just sat down and had a drink of water and then thought that I would sit more comfortably."
"I got my dressing gown on, went downstairs, had a drink of water, went out into the conservatory, went out into the garden. Had a little walk around the garden and I thought: 'Oh, this will ease off.'"

Previous experience
"I knew it was a heart attack because I knew that once you get the pains in the chest and pain in the arm, I knew that it was a heart attack...only because of experience though, you know."

Lay medical knowledge
"Well I'm not an expert, I just have what I have read in the newspapers, but I asked my husband if it could be a heart attack because he had a feeling like ... a belt around [his] chest and down the left arm."—Wife of non-delayer

Intuition
"I knew it was the heart ... does that sound conceited? But you know your own body and I was pretty sure that that was what it was."

Strategy of delayers

Attempts to treat
"Yes I said: 'Oh, you know, I've got this indigestion' and of course my missus says: 'Well take some of your Zantac.' So I did like, you know, but it made no difference and they [mother in law and wife] said: 'Try some lemonade.' Then her mum gave me some mints. I tried everything."

Lay consultation
"He said he thought it could be thyroid but I mean he isn't a doctor ... he said that it could even be a hiatus hernia, because he's got a hiatus hernia and he gets a burning feeling sometimes there."

Use of personal and contextual information
"I had been doing a lot of these fruit inspections so I'd honestly thought it was just working ... but on Friday I'd got home earlier and so I said: 'Ah, I'll do the tea, I'll make something ... .' The only thing I can really do is a fry up stuff and that's what I did. I fried up sausages and got some eggs and got some chips in the oven and we had a fry up ... . So then I just thought: 'Well I've been out drinking, had this fry up and I've got real indigestion.' That's what I thought it was when I went home."

---

of the event. Non-delayers used their experience, medical knowledge, and intuition to reinterpret their symptoms (box).

All of the patients in this group reached a point where they thought they were experiencing either a heart attack or something associated with the heart.

Delayers
The delayers used various medical and non-medical resources to try to bring their symptoms under control. They also consulted lay people and used the information in various ways to try to rationalise the experience of illness. This often resulted in delay as the experience of others had to be compared and discounted. Contextual and personal information was used to reinterpret the situation (box, above).

This process of treatment and continual reassurance and readjustment to the symptoms delayed the realisation that the symptoms were serious enough to require urgent medical intervention. None of the patients in this group considered that they were having a heart attack but eventually came to realise that they were experiencing something serious.

Extended delayers
The extended delayers tried treatments and movement as well as seeking both lay and medical consultation in their attempts to deal with their experience. The greater the number of interventions used, whether in the form of drugs or consultation, the greater the delay. Notable in this group was the influence of contact with the medical profession. Elements of diagnosis by health professionals that discounted patients' risk of having a heart attack and attributed symptoms to other causes both before and during the cardiac event considerably influenced decision making and added to the delay (box, next page).

Patients in this group failed to obtain effective help in managing their symptoms and were eventually admitted to hospital because they could no longer cope.

Extended delayers: two case histories

Case 37

A patient initially thought that her symptoms were caused by a viral infection:

"I thought it's not angina because it's both arms. I mean you think, you tend to kid yourself about these things, and I thought: 'Well my heart doesn't feel as if its palpitating, doing this' [hand gestures]. And you think these things, and I thought well, I thought it could be a viral infection because of these glands coming up. And sweating like a pig as well."

She subsequently contacted her general practitioner's out of hours service and the doctor assured her over the telephone that the symptoms were viral: " 'Oh there's a lot of that going around, it's a viral infection, just take some aspirin and if you're not better after 48 hours ring us up again.' " She therefore believed that her problem was viral and treated it accordingly for nearly 24 hours in spite of worsening symptoms.

Case 43

A patient became progressively short of breath and developed a "severe" indigestion-type pain. He visited his doctor, who diagnosed hiatus hernia and prescribed drug treatment. He did not gain relief from his symptoms and began to experience other symptoms. Having read the information sheet accompanying the drug to treat hiatus hernia, however, he attributed his additional symptoms to side effects from the drug.

"Friday morning [I] was out doing some jobs on the tractor because it was wet, and I went to move and it felt as if I had got grease on the bottom of my shoe. It didn't want to go where I wanted it to. So I went indoors and that and sat down for a little while, looked on the tablet packet and it said there are side effects, that it affects your muscles. So, OK, I wasn't worried—carried on working."

Perception of risk and of heart attacks before the event

Patients' previous perceptions of their own risk varied among the three groups, with more than twice as many of the non-delayers considering themselves to be potentially at risk of a cardiac event compared with the other two groups. In describing a typical potential victim of a heart attack, informants described a stereotype unlike themselves (box, above right).

For most informants their experience of a heart attack differed considerably from their concept of what a heart attack would be like. Heart attacks were thought to be dramatic, sudden events, as often portrayed on television. Informants associated heart attacks with collapse and death, whereas they were, in many cases, still able to function to some degree (box, below right).

Discussion

Studies of patient behaviour and decision making at the time of a heart attack have identified socioeconomic class, education, age, sex, marital status, and race as factors implicated in delay.[4][5] Other variables identified include clinical factors such as having had a heart attack before and the intensity of symptoms.[6][7] Our study used a qualitative approach to explain delay rather than produce statistically representative factors associated with delay.

Perception of heart attack victim and heart attacks

Typical victim

• "Well, yes, there is a sort of stereotypical person—people propping up the bar, swilling beer down, then eating pizza or fish and chips in between cigarettes—I suppose."—Relative of non-delayer

• "If I see someone smoking, drinking, obese, I think 'God, you're in for a heart attack chummy.' "—Delayer

• "My opinion is that it is the guy that's on the dole, sits in front of the TV all day, drinking pints of beer and lager and eating fish and chips. Of course, that's not me!"—Extended delayer

Typical heart attack

• "People going 'aahh' and dying, basically."—Delayer

• "You know, I would have thought somebody clutching, although he [her husband] was clutching but basically just dropping down, you know. The pains and on the floor and not actually being able to do anything."—Wife of non-delayer

• "Well, having heard of people who've had a heart attack, it didn't seem that serious. It seemed as if a heart attack was more of a serious thing ... you've only got seconds to live sort of thing."—Non-delayer

Portrayal in media

• "Well, I saw Superman, you know, when he clutched his chest, went to his arm, and then he died .... Do you remember that, when Superman's adopted father on earth died of a heart attack?"—Delayer

Socioeconomic group and previous occurrence of a heart attack were similar in the three groups, but the age and sex distributions varied, with a greater proportion of men under 65 being non-delayers.

The most critical factor influencing the time taken between onset of symptoms and seeking medical help is that patients and others recognise the symptoms as cardiac in origin. Our results show that intervention could take place at various points in the process to help symptom recognition and speed access to effective treatment. Non-delayers were more likely to see themselves as potentially at risk, were able to describe a wider range of symptoms of a heart attack, and were much less likely to treat their symptoms.

The main focus of information campaigns to date has been to recommend that people experiencing central chest pain (some list additional symptoms) for more than 15 minutes should call an ambulance.[8-10] We found, however, that for most people a heart attack evolved, they experienced the symptoms for much longer than 15 minutes before seeking help, and many were able to contain or relieve their symptoms to some extent. Thus, in most cases, the 15 minute rule may be

Informants' experience of a heart attack

• "Mine wasn't excruciating pain like you hear, you know .... Heart attacks are excruciating and you never forget it ... and falling down with crushing pain, nothing like you've ever had before—in reality it's not like that."—Delayer

• "Er, when she had this heart attack it wasn't the heart attack that I know ... where they lose consciousness and you could give them the kiss of life or something like that. I mean I'd know what to do there, but it wasn't like that you see, you can't give a person the kiss of life if they're not unconscious or they are gasping for breath."—Husband of delayer

• " I mean, I've seen one once, years ago, when I was a coalman. I saw a man have a heart attack. He didn't die on the spot, but he died within an hour or so. He was just on the floor, sort of foaming at the mouth and people milling around him ... but with me, I kept walking, stopping, getting things sorted out, getting back in the car, having a cigarette, driving to a safe location, finding help—nothing like this man."—Extended delayer

| **Key messages** |

- Research using methods that can explain variations in response to cardiac events has been neglected
- Informants in this study thought of heart attacks as sudden dramatic events in which people collapse and probably die, rather than as the evolving event that they experienced
- Those who sought medical help within 4 hours were more likely to see themselves as potentially at risk, knew a wider range of symptoms of a heart attack, and were much less likely to use drugs to treat their symptoms compared with those who waited longer
- Intervention at various points in the decision making process could help recognition of symptoms and speed access to effective treatment

Contributors: AR initiated the research, discussed core ideas, participated in the protocol design, in analysing and interpreting data, and in writing the paper. JC participated in the data collection and in analysing and interpreting data and contributed to the paper. MC participated in the protocol design, discussed core ideas, and contributed to the paper. AR and MC are guarantors for the study.

Funding: This study was funded by the British Heart Foundation.

Conflict of interest: None.

1 Weston CFM, Penny WJ, Julian DG. Guidelines for the early management of patients with myocardial infarction. *BMJ* 1994;308:767-71.
2 Task Force on the Management of Acute Myocardial Infarction of the European Society of Cardiology. Acute myocardial infarction: pre-hospital and in hospital management. *Eur Heart J* 1996;17:43-63.
3 Maycut P, Morehouse R. *Beginning qualitative research—a philosophic and practical guide.* London: Falmer Press, 1994.
4 Hackett TP, Cassem NH. Factors contributing to delay in responding to the signs and symptoms of acute myocardial infarction. *Am J Cardiol* 1969;24:651-8.
5 Schmidt SB, Borsch MA. The pre-hospital phase of acute myocardial infarction in the era of thrombolysis. *Am J Cardiol* 1990;65:1411-5.
6 Weilgosz AT, Nolan RP. Understanding delay in response to symptoms of acute myocardial infarction. *Circulation* 1991;84:2193-5.
7 Heriot AG, Brecker SJ, Coltart DJ. Delay in presentation after myocardial infarction. *J R Soc Med* 1993;86:642-4.
8 East Kent Health Authority. *Home treatment guide.* Canterbury: EKHA, 1996.
9 British Heart Foundation. *Information card.* London: BHF, 1996.
10 Brighton Heart Attack Study. *Heart attack. Action Leaflet.* Brighton: BHAS, 1995.

(Accepted 16 January 1998)

too simplistic to be effective. Linked with this is the stereotypical heart attack victim and the perception of a heart attack as a dramatic event in which people collapse with crushing chest pains and probably die. Clearly, the myth that a heart attack is a dramatic event needs to be dispelled and public perceptions of a heart attack and its associated symptoms need to be changed.

Commentary: Grounded theory and the constant comparative method

Judith Green

Health Services Research Unit, London School of Hygiene and Tropical Medicine, London WC1E 7HT

Judith Green, *lecturer in sociology*

The potential for qualitative research to sensitise policymakers and practitioners to the perceptions of health service users and professionals[1] and to strengthen aetiological and health services research[2] is now well recognised, but the reporting of qualitative data continues to generate dissatisfaction for both researchers and readers. For qualitative researchers used to the more discursive formats of social science journals, the need to present succinctly with clear implications for policy or practice can constrain reports of the theoretical richness, complexity, and ambiguity of their research findings. For readers, small sample sizes and illustrative quotes imply impressionistic accounts of doubtful validity and generalisability. The development of guidelines for producing[3 4] and judging qualitative research[5-7] has been helpful for researchers and editors, but a problem remains for many readers about the credibility of published qualitative research in medical journals. Few authors report how validity and reliability were maximised,[8] and, indeed, such criteria may be inappropriate in theoretical rather than empirical studies, which have traditionally been the most influential in health.[9]

Grounded theory

One strategy used by some researchers to improve the credibility of published papers has been to include routinely the line: "the data were analysed using grounded theory," which suggests an esoteric technique guaranteeing rigour. Unfortunately, what follows may be merely an account of some key themes in the data, with brief textual quotes in illustration, and scep-

tical readers remain unconvinced that qualitative analysis is anything other than journalistic reportage. Ruston et al have used the constant comparative method in a more analytical way to generate data which contribute to understanding what stops people seeking help quickly after a heart attack and also explore patients' perceptions of what a normal heart attack looks like. These findings are most useful to practitioners and health promoters, and the authors have provided information on how they improved reliability. However, the constant comparative method, which is derived from grounded theory, can offer more than this when it is applied and reported well.

Grounded theory was developed by the sociologists Anselm Strauss and Barney Glaser as a way of formalising the operations needed to develop theory from empirical data.[10-12] It is a methodological approach (entailing a cyclical process of induction, deduction, and verification) and a set of strategies of data analysis to improve the reliability and theoretical depth of analysis. Particular attention is paid to the processes entailed in coding data. Too often in published health research coding has meant simply labelling data extracts as examples of themes the researcher was interested in. Coding should entail comparing indicators (such as actions or fragments of text or talk) to refine their fit to underlying concepts. Initial coding can be based on what Glaser and Strauss call in vivo codes as well as on conceptually derived codes. In vivo codes are the categories used by respondents themselves to organise their world—for example, the description of some patients as "normal rubbish" noted by Jeffrey in his work on staff in accident and emergency departments. These were patients attending with minor or self inflicted injuries or those who had social rather than medical problems.[13] However, such codes are provisional and are essentially descriptive summaries of respondents' own accounts. Analytical coding requires also questioning and comparison. Indicators are coded according to a coding paradigm, which the researcher uses to ask a battery of questions of each indicator to establish its properties, its dimensions, and its relation to other codes. Constant comparison of indicators with each other refines their fit to the emerging conceptual categories. In the example of Jeffrey's study of staff in accident and emergency departments,[13] the properties of patients termed normal rubbish were inductively generated through analysing accounts of why staff did not like dealing with certain patients. Coding also has to be theoretically informed: Jeffrey used sociological theory about the sick role to analyse the properties both of patients termed normal rubbish and of "good patients."[13] Normal rubbish were patients whose behaviour did not conform to social norms of the sick role, whereas good patients enabled staff to practise clinical and technical skills.

Validity

The key to developing rigorous and valid theory using the constant comparative method is the search for deviant cases. These can be within the researcher's data, which are searched for exceptions to the emerging relations between codes. Grounded theory also advocates theoretical sampling, in which potentially deviant cases can be purposively sampled as the study progresses. A full report of qualitative analysis should account for deviant cases and how they have contributed to refining theory. Constant comparison does not stop within the researcher's own data set. Theoretical insight and comparative material comes from other research, perhaps outside the substantive field of interest.

For Glaser and Strauss social phenomena are always complex and require sensitive and dense theory to account for as much variation in the data as possible. The challenge for qualitative researchers is to find ways of reflecting this complexity. To do this they need adequate methods of analysis to offer complex theoretical insights within the constraints of biomedical and health services journals. Without such endeavour, qualitative research will remain descriptive anecdote.

1 Fitzpatrick R, Boulton M. Qualitative methods for assessing health care. *Quality in Health Care* 1994;3:107-13.
2 Black N. Why we need qualitative research. *J Epidemiol Community Health* 1994;48:425-6.
3 Mays N, Pope C. Rigour and qualitative research. *BMJ* 1995;311:109-12.
4 Seale C, Silverman D. Ensuring rigour in qualitative research. *Eur J Public Health* 1997;7:379-84.
5 Blaxter M. Criteria for the evaluation of qualitative research papers. *Medical Sociology News* 1996;22(1):68-71.
6 Boulton M, Fitzpatrick R. Evaluating qualitative research. *Evidence Based Health Policy and Management* 1997;1:83-5.
7 Dowell J, Huby G, Smith C, eds. *Scottish consensus statement on qualitative research in primary health care.* Dundee: Tayside Centre for General Practice, 1995.
8 Boulton M, Fitzpatrick R, Swinburn C. Qualitative research in health care. II. A structured review and evaluation of studies. *Journal of Evaluation in Clinical Practice* 1996;2:171-9.
9 Chard JA, Lilford RJ, Court BV. Qualitative medical sociology: what are its crowning achievements? *J R Soc Med* 1997;90:604-9.
10 Glaser B, Strauss A. *The discovery of grounded theory.* Chicago: Aldine Publishing, 1967.
11 Strauss A. *Qualitative analysis for social scientists.* Cambridge: Cambridge University Press, 1987.
12 Strauss A, Corbin J. *Basics of qualitative research: grounded theory procedures and techniques.* London: Sage, 1990.
13 Jeffrey, R. Normal rubbish: deviant patients in casualty departments. *Sociology of Health and Illness* 1979;1:90-108.

Qualitative research and evidence based medicine

Judith Green, Nicky Britten

Health Services
Research Unit,
London School of
Hygiene and
Tropical Medicine,
London
WC1E 7HT
Judith Green,
lecturer in sociology

Department of
General Practice,
United Medical and
Dental School of
Guy's and
St Thomas's
Hospitals, London
SE11 6SP
Nicky Britten,
*senior lecturer in
medical sociology*

Correspondence to:
Dr Green
j.green@lshtm.
ac.uk

BMJ 1998;316:1230-2

Qualitative research may seem unscientific and anecdotal to many medical scientists. However, as the critics of evidence based medicine are quick to point out, medicine itself is more than the application of scientific rules.[1] Clinical experience, based on personal observation, reflection, and judgment, is also needed to translate scientific results into treatment of individual patients.[2] Personal experience is often characterised as being anecdotal, ungeneralisable, and a poor basis for making scientific decisions. However, it is often a more powerful persuader than scientific publication in changing clinical practice,[3-5] as illustrated by the occasional series "A patient who changed my practice" in the *BMJ*.[6]

In an attempt to widen the scope of evidence based medicine, recent workshops have included units on other subjects, including economic analysis and qualitative research.[7] However, to do so is to move beyond the discipline of clinical epidemiology that underpins evidence based medicine. Qualitative research, in particular, addresses research questions that are different from those considered by clinical epidemiology. Qualitative research can investigate practitioners' and patients' attitudes, beliefs, and preferences, and the whole question of how evidence is turned into practice. The value of qualitative methods lies in their ability to pursue systematically the kinds of research questions that are not easily answerable by experimental methods.

We use the example of asthma treatment to illustrate how qualitative methods can broaden the scope of evidence based medicine. Although there is consensus over evidence based practice in the treatment of asthma,[8] questions remain about general practitioners' use of clinical guidelines and patients' use of prescribed medication.[9]

Naturalism

Various qualitative methods are used in health research, but they share some basic orientations (see box).[10] The first is a commitment to naturalism, or understanding health behaviour in its everyday context. Results of drug trials may inform practitioners about the optimum effects of therapeutic agents, but even pragmatic trials are not the same as everyday experience. For instance, in today's highly competitive workplace, some people report that they need to seem "healthy" at work and do not want to be seen taking medications.[11][12] Thus, appearances may be more important to some people than symptom relief.

Summary points

Qualitative methods can help bridge the gap between scientific evidence and clinical practice

Qualitative research findings provide rigorous accounts of treatment regimens in everyday contexts

This can help us understand the barriers to using evidence based medicine, and its limitations in informing decisions about treatment

Recognising the limits of evidence based medicine does not imply a rejection of research evidence but awareness that different research questions require different kinds of research

Interpretation

A second aim of most qualitative studies is that of interpretation: investigating how patients and practitioners make sense of "objective" variables such as peak flow readings. Subjective meanings are crucial to an understanding of how treatment regimens integrate with everyday life. For instance, Adams et al found that half of the asthmatic people they interviewed did not see themselves as asthma sufferers.[12] Their "bad chests" were perceived as an acute and temporary problem, better treated with drugs to relieve the symptoms than daily prophylactic medication.

Various strategies that enable asthma sufferers to continue "normal" everyday life, despite symptoms that health professionals would see as objectively problematic, have been reported. Adams et al cite avoidance of triggers such as sexual intercourse, physical exertion, or spending time outdoors in the summer.[12] Although these adaptive strategies might seem extreme, patients interpret alternatives, such as using daily preventative medication, as accepting a stigmatising label of "asthmatic." Thus, findings about patients' possible interpretations of symptoms are essential to understanding likely medication use.

Process

The third contribution of qualitative studies to the evidence base on asthma is the assumption that social life is a process, and that interventions and the changes

Originally published in *BMJ* 1998; **316**: 180–83.

> **Basic orientations of qualitative methods**
>
> • Naturalism—understanding treatment regimens in an everyday context
> • Interpretation—what meaning do symptoms and treatment regimens have for patients and practitioners?
> • Process—how might these meanings change over time?
> • Interaction—how does communication between patients and practitioners impact on the meaning of medication?
> • Relativism—scientific "reality" may look different from different perspectives

they bring have to be accommodated within the patient's "biography."[15] Patients with asthma may have to manage medication over a whole lifetime, rather than for the limited duration of even a long drug trial, and integrate an "asthmatic" identity into their other social roles. As the study by Adams et al suggests, for many patients this will involve taking control of their medication, and limiting contact with professionals.[12] Conrad's classic study of compliance with medication showed that patients with epilepsy often "tested" themselves to see if their epilepsy had resolved by taking themselves off medication completely or for short periods of time.[14] People with asthma also have to integrate symptoms and their management with both the practicalities of everyday life and the psychological "self" over time.[12]

Interaction and relativism

Qualitative studies often take interaction as a focus of research, rather than a given factor. Katon and Kleinman viewed encounters between doctors and their patients as the bringing together of often conflicting explanatory systems about health and illness, which required negotiation to achieve good outcomes.[15] The medical interview may be a meeting between very different views of reality.[16] Qualitative sociologists have shown the value of a relativist approach, that focuses on these different explanatory systems.

Attitudes and adherence

One illustration of this from published reports on adherence is general attitudes to medication. Although one "reality" is that medication for asthma reduces morbidity and mortality, and can benefit users with few costs to their everyday lives, qualitative studies suggest a rather different "reality" for patients. Firstly, there is evidence that some patients have negative views about medicines, regarding these as unnatural substances that diminish the body's own ability to fight disease and cause dependence.[17] Many doctors, however, make the commonsense assumption that patients are seeking medication.[18] This general finding is borne out in specific studies of patients with asthma.[19] These studies show that patients worry about becoming physically and psychologically dependent on bronchodilators, and have even more deep seated worries about the long term effects of inhaled corticosteroids.[11] Regarding patients' views of reality as ignorant or misguided

and attempting to persuade them of the value of a biomedical approach have limited value in increasing adherence, and the need to integrate patients' perspectives has been recognised recently.[15 20 21]

Assessing qualitative research

These orientations of naturalism, interpretation, process, interaction, and relativism may be shared by commonsense accounts of medical practice, such as the personal anecdote. There are, however, important differences between anecdotes (stories told for their dramatic or other qualities, without analysis or critical evaluation) and qualitative research. Rigorously conducted qualitative research is based on explicit sampling strategies, systematic analysis of data, and a commitment to examining counter explanations. Ideally, methods should be transparent, allowing the reader to assess the validity and the extent to which results might be applicable to their own clinical practice. The generalisability of qualitative research is likely to be conceptual rather than numerical.[22] The studies discussed here, for instance, provide evidence for a number of conceptual issues such as the links between denial of the diagnosis of asthma and medication use or the importance of generally negative views about medication. For the practitioner, the value of these findings is that they are sensitised to issues which could usefully be explored with patients. A number of guidelines now exist to aid both journal editors and readers in assessing qualitative health research.[10 23-25]

Conclusion

The argument that qualitative research can contribute answers to questions not easily addressed by randomised controlled trials is not new. Much has been written on the uses and value of sociology for medicine, and indeed there has been a growing acceptance of its methods in healthcare research, including its contribution to randomised controlled trials when these are appropriate.[26] However, in the context of the debate about evidence based medicine, it is vital to reiterate that good "evidence" goes further than the results of meta-analysis of randomised controlled trials. The

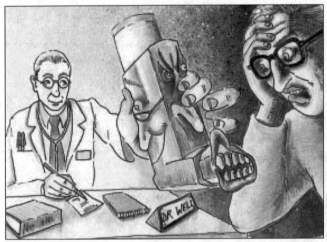

limitations of these trials, and the evidence about barriers to their utilisation by practitioners, should not lead to cynicism about the role of research evidence in health care. We need to be sure that it is the right kind of research to answer the questions posed.

Funding: No additional funding.
Conflict of interest: None.

1 Naylor CD. Grey zones of clinical practice: some limits to evidence-based medicine. *Lancet* 1995;345:840-2.
2 Freidson E. *Profession of medicine: a study of the sociology of applied knowledge.* New York: Dodd, Mead and Company, 1970.
3 Atkinson P. *Medical talk and medical work: the liturgy of the clinic.* London: Sage, 1995.
4 Greer A. The state of the art versus the state of the science. *Int J Technol Assess Health Care* 1988;4:5-26.
5 Greer A. Scientific knowledge and social consensus. *Controlled Clin Trials* 1994;15:431-6.
6 Burdett-Smith P. A patient who changed my practice: always check the respiratory rate. *BMJ* 1997;314:1549.
7 Unit for Evidence Based Practice and Policy. *Fourth UK workshop on teaching evidence-based practice study pack.* London: University College London Medical School, 1997.
8 British Thoracic Society and others. Guidelines for the management of asthma: a summary. *BMJ* 1993;306:776-82.
9 Audit Commission. *What the doctor ordered: a study of GP fundholders in England and Wales.* London: HMSO, 1996.
10 Mays N, Pope C, eds. *Qualitative research in health care.* London: BMJ Publishing Group, 1996.
11 Hewett G. *"Just a part of me": men's reflections on chronic asthma.* London: South Bank University, 1994. (Occasional papers in sociology and social policy.)
12 Adams S, Pill R, Jones A. Medication, chronic illness and identity: the perspective of people with asthma. *Soc Sci Med* 1997;45:189-201.
13 Bury M. Chronic illness as biographical disruption. *Sociology of Health and Illness* 1982;4:167-82.
14 Conrad P. The meaning of medications: another look at compliance. *Soc Sci Med* 1985;20:29-37.
15 Katon W, Kleinman A. Doctor-patient negotiation and other social science strategies in patient care. In: Eisenberg L, Kleinman A, eds. *The relevance of social science to medicine.* Dordrecht: Reidel, 1981.
16 Mishler EG. *The discourse of medicine: dialectics of medical interviews.* Norwood, NJ: Ablex, 1984.
17 Britten N. Patients' ideas about medicines: a qualitative study in a general practice population *Br J Gen Pract* 1994;44:465-8.
18 Hull FM, Marshall T. Sources of information about new drugs and attitudes towards drug prescribing: an international study of differences between primary care physicians. *Fam Pract* 1987;4:123-8.
19 Osman LM, Russell IT, Friend JAR, Legge JS, Douglas JG. Predicting patient attitudes to asthma medication. *Thorax* 1993;48:827-30.
20 Marinker M. Writing prescriptions is easy. *BMJ* 1997;314:747-8.
21 Tuckett D, Boulton M, Olson C, Williams A. *Meetings between experts: an approach to sharing ideas in medical consultations.* London: Tavistock, 1985.
22 Fitzpatrick R, Boulton M. Qualitative methods for assessing health care. *Quality in Health Care* 1994;3:107-113.
23 Dowell J, Huby G, Smith C, eds. *Scottish consensus statement on qualitative research in primary health care.* Dundee: Tayside Centre for General Practice, 1995.
24 Boulton M, Fitzpatrick R, Swinburn C. Qualitative research in health care. II. A structured review and evaluation of studies. *J Eval Clin Pract* 1996;2:171-9.
25 Blaxter M. Criteria for the evaluation of qualitative research papers. *Med Sociol News* 1996;22:68-71.
26 Oakley A. Who's afraid of the randomised controlled trial? Some dilemmas of the scientific method and good research practice. In: *Women's health counts.* London: Routledge, 1990.

(Accepted 21 November 1997)

Papers that analyse very rare events (case control studies)

BACKGROUND

It is not ethically possible to do randomised controlled trials into the effect of an agent that is thought to cause harm. We must look at those who have already come to harm and analyse their past to look for exposure to possible harmful agents. The control group in this type of study is made up of individuals that have not come to harm. Evaluating such *case control studies* requires different questions from those we generally ask about randomised controlled trials but the principle of addressing the sampling frame, potential biases and confounding factors, and relevance of results is the same.

SUGGESTED AIM FOR THIS SESSION

For participants to develop, and feel confident in helping others to develop, the ability to determine whether the results and conclusions of a research article which incriminates (or exonerates) a putative harmful agent are valid and applicable to their own practice.

SUGGESTED LEARNING OBJECTIVES FOR THIS SESSION

By the end of this session, participants should be able to:
● establish whether a case control study addressed an important and relevant question;
● assess the methodological quality of the study using a structured checklist;
● assess the significance of the results in terms of the magnitude and precision of the estimate of harm;
● comment critically on the application and implementation of the results.

SET ARTICLE

Cesar JA, Victora CG, Barros FC, Santos IS, Flores JA. Impact of breast feeding on admission for pneumonia during postneonatal period in Brazil: nested case control study. *BMJ* 1999; **318**: 1316–20.

Clinical scenario

Dr Ashok Sawar is a consultant paediatrician working in a community hospital in a remote rural area of Gujerat, north India. The local catchment population is largely poor tenant farmers, with a low level of literacy and an infant mortality rate of 42 per 1000. Although this rate is gradually falling, Dr Sawar notes that there have recently been two deaths from pneumonia in infants under 12 weeks of age who (unusually for this population) had been exclusively bottle fed. He decides to explore the hypothesis that bottle feeding had increased the infants' risk of serious respiratory problems and while searching the literature, finds the article reprinted here.

SUGGESTIONS FOR GROUP EXERCISES

When you have read the paper, try one or more of the following.

1. A role play in which Dr Sawar and a group of midwives and community health workers discuss the findings and the implications for health education initiatives.
2. A teaching situation in which some final-year medical or nursing students are asked to appraise the paper and express concern that the findings are "only applicable to Brazil".

SUGGESTION FOR INDIVIDUAL STUDY

First, complete the critical appraisal checklist. Note that in this article the putative "harmful event" is a negative one, i.e. *not* breast feeding. Consider the concerns of the students in the second group exercise above. Decide what your own concerns are about the generalisability of these findings to Gujerat, India. Construct a literature search to see if you can identify additional potentially relevant papers. Assuming you find nothing that casts serious doubts on the generalisability of these findings, compose a letter to a hypothetical Minister of Health in India asking for a review of government policy on the advertising of formula milk in poor rural areas.

CRITICAL APPRAISAL CHECKLIST FOR AN ARTICLE DESCRIBING A CASE CONTROL STUDY

Note that the questions on the checklist are really looking for problems of bias, confounding, low power, and poor validity.

A. Are the results of the trial valid and do they contain minimum bias?	Yes/No/Don't know
1. Did the study address a clearly focused question (PEO)? • Population • Exposure to risk factor(s) over specified time period • Outcome(s)	
2. Were the authors interested in very uncommon or rare *outcomes*? (Not rare exposures; examining rare outcomes is the main justification for conducting a case control study)	
3. Was the case control study "population based"[1] (stronger) or not (weaker)?	
4. Aside from the outcome of interest, were the two groups (cases and controls) similar in other important factors at the start of the study (e.g. sex, age, social class)?	
5. Were there four or fewer controls matched to each case?	
B. What are the results?	
6. How large was the effect of the exposure? • What outcomes were measured? (Measures of risk: odds ratio [similar to relative risk when the outcome is rare])[2]	
7. How precise was the estimate of the exposure effect? • What are its confidence limits (or p-values)?	
C. How relevant are the results?	
8. Were the study participants sufficiently different from my population that this study doesn't help me at all?	

[1] Population-based case control studies take into account and may include *all* the cases in a defined population, usually identified from some kind of disease register. This minimises the selection bias that plagues non-population based case control studies.

[2] Case control studies cannot give true measures of relative risk, because their authors do not know the population base (denominator of relative risk) from which the cases and controls are drawn. Therefore, they usually cite odds ratios, which approximate the relative risk so long as the outcome of interest (defining a case) is very uncommon or rare. Odds ratios (and case control studies) of outcomes that are not very uncommon or rare should be viewed with caution.

FURTHER READING

Donald A, Greenhalgh T. *A hands-on guide to evidence-based health care: practice and implementation.* Oxford: Blackwell Science, 1999.

Greenhalgh T. *How to read a paper: the basics of evidence based medicine.* London: BMJ Books, 1997. See in particular Chapter 4: Assessing methodological quality, pages 53–68.

Levine M, Walter S, Lee H, Haines T, Holbrook A, Moyer V. Users' guides to the medical literature. IV. How to use an article about harm. *JAMA* 1994; **271**: 1615–19.

Impact of breast feeding on admission for pneumonia during postneonatal period in Brazil: nested case-control study

Juraci A César, Cesar G Victora, Fernando C Barros, Iná S Santos, José A Flores

Editorial by Latham

Departamento Materno Infantil, Fundação Universidade do Rio Grande, Rio Grande do Sol, Brazil Juraci A César, *assistant professor*

Departamento de Medicina Social, Universidade Federal de Pelotas, Rio Grande do Sol Cesar G Victora, *professor*

Fernando C Barros, *professor*

Iná S Santos, *associate professor*

continued over

BMJ 1999;318:1316–20

Abstract

Objective To determine whether breast feeding protects infants against pneumonia and whether the protection varies with age.

Design Nested case-control study.

Setting Pelotas, southern Brazil.

Subjects Cases were 152 infants aged 28-364 days who had been admitted to hospital for pneumonia. Controls were 2391 cases in a population based case-control study.

Main outcome measure Odds ratio of admission for pneumonia according to type of milk consumed (breast milk alone, breast and formula milk, or formula milk and other fluids only), use of fluid supplements apart from formula milk, and use of solid supplements.

Results Infants who were not being breast fed were 17 times more likely than those being breast fed without formula milk to be admitted to hospital for pneumonia (95% confidence interval 7.7 to 36.0). This relative risk was 61 (19.0 to 195.5) for children under 3 months old, decreasing to 10 (2.8 to 36.2) thereafter. Supplementation with solids was associated with a relative risk of 13.4 (7.6 to 23.5) for all infants and 175 (21.8 to 1405.1) for those under 3 months old.

Conclusion Breast feeding protects young children against pneumonia, especially in the first months of life. These results may be used for targeting intervention campaigns at the most vulnerable age groups.

Introduction

Pneumonia is the leading cause of death in children under 5 years old worldwide,[1][2] and breast milk is the most important food in the first year of life.[3]

Several studies in less developed countries have assessed the effect of breast feeding on the risk of developing acute lower respiratory infections, particularly pneumonia.[4] Most of these studies show a protective effect of breast milk on pneumonia, but causality has not yet been shown.[4] In addition, whether this protection changes with age, as has been shown for diarrhoea,[5] is not known.

We performed a nested case-control study in southern Brazil to assess whether breast feeding protects young children against pneumonia and whether this protection varies with age.

Participants and methods

Study population

Throughout 1993 all women who lived in urban areas and had their babies in Pelotas, southern Brazil, were interviewed soon after delivery in the city's hospital. Over 99% of all births in this city take place in such hospitals.[6] A systematic sample of 655 newborn infants was selected for home visiting at 1 and 3 months of age according to date and time of birth. In the first month the mothers of 99.1% (5256) of the children were interviewed and in the third month 98.3% (5214). These infants were also visited at the age of 6 months. As additional funds were obtained for data collection, the sampling fraction was increased to 1144, including the 655 visited at 1 and 3 months of age. These samples represent 12.3% (655) of all children from the original cohort in the first and third months and 21.6% (1144) in the sixth.

Defining cases

Cases of pneumonia were identified through daily visits to the city's hospitals. Children who were born in 1993 and had been admitted to a hospital when aged 28-364 days were considered for inclusion in the study. Two independent referees (paediatricians) reviewed all the available information on each child from hospital's records. Pneumonia was diagnosed from the presence of all clinical signs (difficult or rapid breathing, chest indrawing), presence of rales, and—whenever available—results of laboratory and radiological tests. Whenever the two referees disagreed, a third senior referee established the final diagnosis.

Defining controls

The control group was made up of children taking part in the cohort study. For cases aged 28-89 days, controls were infants at the first home visit, who were aged about 30 days. For cases aged 90-179 days, controls were infants at the second home visit, and for cases aged 180-364 days, controls were infants at the third visit.

For each interview all available controls were used. The study was therefore ratified for age but not matched at the individual level. A child who became a case at, say, 9 months old should have been a control at an earlier age. This characterises this study as a case base, or inclusive, design.[7]

Questionnaire

The mothers of cases were interviewed at home soon after the infant had been discharged from hospital using the same questionnaire as was used for the mothers of controls. Information on diet was collected for cases at the age of their corresponding controls at the home visit. For example, for a case aged 45 days dietary information was obtained for the exact age of 30 days. Three variables were studied.

• Type of milk consumed—breast milk alone, breast and formula milk, or other fluids alone (water, teas, juices, formula milk, or any other liquid supplement except breast milk; this group was considered to be completely weaned)

Originally published in *BMJ* 1999; **318**: 1316–20.

- Use of fluid supplements—whether infants received water, teas, juices, or any other liquid supplements excluding formula milk
- Use of solid and semisolid supplements.

Social class was based on family income, parental schooling, the occupation of the head of household (person with highest salary). This resulted in the following categories: bourgeois and new small bourgeois (professionals and owners of large businesses), small traditional bourgeois (owners of small businesses and shopkeepers), atypical proletariat (non-manual workers in regular employment), typical proletariat (manual workers in regular employment), and subproletariat (unemployed and casual workers).[8] Family income was defined as the total amount received by all people who lived in the one home during the previous month. This total was converted into the number of minimum wages.

Sample size

The sample size studied was sufficient for detecting an odds ratio of 2.0 for exposures present in 25% of the control children, with an α error of 0.05 and a power of 80%.[9] An additional 40% was added to adjust for confounding variables and to compensate for possible refusals.[10] According to this estimate, the final sample size should have at least 143 cases and 572 controls (four controls per case).

Statistical analysis

We measured odds ratios with 95% confidence intervals and used the χ^2 test for contingency tables in analyses.[11] We adjusted analyses using unconditional multiple logistic regression according to a previously determined hierarchical framework (figure). In this model some variables are assumed to mediate their effects through other variables as well as directly. The outcome variable was admission for pneumonia. The significance level for the inclusion of each variable in the model was measured by the likelihood ratio test. The final model included all variables that had a P value up to 0.10 after adjustment for variables in the same and higher levels of the framework. In addition, each ordinal variable—for example, family income group—was evaluated for linear tendency. When this association was significant and did not deviate from linearity, the variable was included in the model as a linear component. When missing values were less than 5% of all cases, they were recorded as the mode. Data on social class were missing in 7% of interviews,[12] and we therefore created a separate category for missing values for this variable. All data were analysed with SPSS for Windows[13] and Egret.[14]

Results

Of the 5304 infants in the original cohort, 152 (2.9%) were admitted to a hospital with pneumonia in the postneonatal period.

Among 250 variables tested, only social class, family income, and maternal schooling, age, parity, and weight gained during pregnancy were associated with outcome (table 1).

Table 2 shows the frequency distributions of cases and controls according to these variables. The fact that there were more controls aged 6-11 months was due to the sampling scheme used in the cohort study. This does not affect the analyses since all information on feeding was referred to the exact age at the start of each age range.[7]

Level	Variable
First	Sex and social class
Second	Family income, maternal schooling, and paternal schooling
Third	Maternal age, parity, and intrapartum interval
Fourth	Weight gained during pregnancy
Fifth	Preterm and intrauterine growth retardation
Sixth	Consumption of milk, other fluids, and solid and semisolid supplements
Outcome	Admission for pneumonia

Hierarchical framework for multiple logistic regression

Hospital Pediátrico Santo Antônio, Porto Alegre, Rio Grande do Sol

José A Flores, *senior radiologist*

Correspondence to: Professor J A César, Maternal and Child Epidemiology Unit, London School of Hygiene and Tropical Medicine, 49-51 Bedford Square, London WC1B 3DP juraci.cesar@lshtm.ac.uk

Table 3 shows that the relative risk of admission for pneumonia for infants receiving breast and formula milk or other fluids alone was 3.8 and 16.7 respectively in comparison with infants who were exclusively breast fed. When infants who received fluid supplements were compared with those who did not the risk disappeared after adjusted analysis. Infants receiving solid and semisolid supplements had a relative risk of 8.5 of being admitted in comparison with those who did not receive such supplements.

Table 1 Unconditional multiple logistic regression model for risk of postneonatal pneumonia

Variable	Odds ratio (95% CI)
Model 1: sex	
Male	1.16 (0.84 to 1.60)
Female	1.00
P value	0.36
Model 2: model 1+social class*	
Bourgeois and new small bourgeois	0.20 (0.27 to 1.44)
Small traditional bourgeois	1.49 (0.89 to 2.47)
Atypical proletariat	1.00
Typical proletariat	1.78 (1.14 to 2.76)
Subproletariat	3.50 (2.15 to 5.70)
P value for linear trend	<0.001
Model 3: model 2+maternal schooling+family income	
Maternal schooling (years):	
0	2.70 (0.98 to 7.45)
1 4	3.24 (1.73 to 6.09)
5 8	1.97 (1.07 to 3.61)
≥9	1.00
P value for linear trend	<0.001
Model 4: model 3+maternal age+parity	
Maternal age (years):	
<20	1.98 (1.12 to 3.51)
20 24	1.32 (0.82 to 2.13)
25 29	1.00
30 34	0.96 (0.56 to 1.63)
≥35	0.75 (0.40 to 1.42)
P value for linear trend	0.08
Parity:	
0	1.00
1	1.05 (0.64 to 1.74)
2	1.53 (0.87 to 2.68)
≥3	2.86 (1.64 to 4.99)
P value for linear trend	<0.01
Model 5: model 4+weight gained during pregnancy	
Weight gained during pregnancy	
<10 kg	1.38 (1.00 to 1.92)
≥10 kg	1.00
P value	0.05

*Bourgeois and new small bourgeois are equivalent to professionals and owners of large businesses, small traditional bourgeois to owners of small businesses and shopkeepers, atypical proletariat to non manual workers in regular employment, typical proletariat to manual workers in regular employment, and subproletariat to unemployed and casual workers.

Table 2 Numbers (percentages) of cases of pneumonia and controls according to main risk factors

Risk factor	Cases (n=152)	Controls (n=2391)
Sex:		
Male	81 (53)	1197 (50)
Female	71 (47)	1194 (50)
Age (days):		
30-89	47 (31)	649 (27)
90-179	62 (41)	644 (27)
180-364	43 (28)	1098 (46)
Social class*:		
Bourgeois (all categories)	26 (17)	499 (21)
Atypical proletariat	39 (26)	1034 (43)
Typical proletariat	42 (27)	518 (22)
Subproletariat	30 (20)	174 (7)
Family income (No of minimum wages per month†):		
≤1	34 (22)	415 (17)
1.1-3	72 (47)	1103 (46)
>3	46 (30)	873 (36)
Maternal schooling (years):		
0	6 (4)	63 (3)
1-4	67 (44)	557 (23)
5-8	65 (43)	1153 (48)
≥9	14 (9)	618 (26)
Maternal age (years):		
<20	35 (23)	358 (15)
20-24	41 (27)	719 (30)
25-29	35 (23)	633 (26)
30-34	26 (17)	438 (18)
≥35	15 (10)	243 (10)
Parity:		
0	42 (28)	849 (35)
1	30 (20)	663 (28)
2	26 (17)	465 (19)
≥3	54 (35)	414 (17)
Weight gained during pregnancy:		
<10 kg	82 (54)	1584 (66)
≥10 kg	70 (46)	807 (34)

*Bourgeois (all categories) includes professionals, owners of large businesses, owners of small businesses, and shopkeepers; atypical proletariat is equivalent to non-manual workers in regular employment, typical proletariat to manual workers in regular employment, and subproletariat to unemployed and casual workers.
†Around $100 in 1993.

Table 4 shows that after adjustment infants receiving breast and formula milk at the age of 1-2.9 months were 2.9 times more likely to be admitted for pneumonia than were those who received breast milk alone. The relative risk for infants who were completely weaned was 61.1. From age 3-5.9 months these relative risks were 3.4 and to 10.1 respectively. From age 6-11.9 months the odds ratios were 3.7 and 9.2 respectively. The interaction between age and the type of milk consumed was significant (P < 0.001).

Table 3 Odds ratios for developing pneumonia according to type of food given

Variable	Cases (n=152)	Controls (n=2391)	Odds ratio (95% CI)*	
			Crude	Adjusted†
Type of milk consumed				
Breast milk alone	9	779	1.0	1.0
Breast and formula milk	23	563	4.5 (2.1 to 9.9)	3.8 (1.7 to 8.9)
Other fluids alone (completely weaned)	120	1049	19.0 (9.3 to 38.7)	16.7 (7.7 to 36.0)
P value			<0.001	<0.001
Fluid supplementation				
Fluids given	149	2230	4.5 (1.4 to 14.5)	1.3 (0.3 to 4.9)
Fluids not given	3	161	1.0	1.0
P value			<0.001	0.73
Solid and semisolid supplementation				
Supplements given	97	1226	13.4 (7.6 to 23.5)	8.5 (4.7 to 15.4)
Supplements not given	55	1165	1.0	1.0
P value			<0.001	<0.001

*Stratified by age groups of 1-2.9, 3-5.9, and 6-11.9 months.
†For sex, social class, family income, and maternal schooling, age, parity, and weight gained during pregnancy. In addition, each feeding variable was controlled for the other two.

The crude analysis showed that the risk associated with the intake of supplementary foods in the first months was 175 for children aged 1-2.9 months, 9.1 for children aged 3-5.9 months, and 0.7 for children aged 6-11.9 months. The odds ratio of pneumonia admission for all children who received supplementary food was 13.4.

Discussion

Methodological limitations

Case-control studies may be affected by several biases.[4] [15-18] Reverse causality bias—that is, repeated respiratory illnesses leading to a change in breastfeeding pattern—was avoided by regarding as still breastfed infants who had stopped breast feeding because of a respiratory infection up to two months before admission. Another possibility is recall bias, since mothers of cases in a given age range (1-2.9, 3-5.9, and 6-11.9 months) were asked to provide retrospective information on feeding patterns at the beginning of that interval, while mothers of control children were interviewed within a few days of that date. To assess how this could affect the estimates of relative risk we analysed the reported feeding patterns of 32 infants who had been both a case and a control. For 26 infants the type of milk consumed was the same in both interviews (three were receiving breast milk alone, five were receiving breast and formula milk, and 18 were completely weaned). The kappa index was 0.81, reflecting good concordance. Of the six mothers whose information was discordant, five overestimated and one underestimated the intake of breast milk. With this adjustment the odds ratio for breast and formula milk increased from 3.5 to 5.6 and that for formula milk decreased from 9.9 to 6.9 (table 5). Therefore, recall bias may have reduced the estimate of risk for children receiving both breast and formula milk and increased the risk for infants who had been completely weaned. However, our main conclusions remain unchanged. Berkson paradox was controlled for during adjusted analysis,[19] and limitation related to diagnostic criteria was reduced by using referees.[12]

Previous studies

Recent publications have emphasised the need for using standard definitions of feeding patterns to allow comparison between studies.[20] In our sample few infants were exclusively breast fed—20% in the first month and 1.6% at three months—because formula milk and herbal teas are widely used.[21] The low rate of exclusive breast feeding precludes the use of such infants as the baseline category with the lowest expected risk. We therefore used three different variables (type of milk consumed, intake of fluid supplements, and intake of solid and semisolid supplements) to characterise feeding patterns. With this approach the dose-response effect of the type of milk consumed could be assessed—most studies treat breast feeding as a dichotomous variable[4] [18]—and the effects of milk, fluids, and other foods could be separated.

Several studies from less developed countries show that the risk of acquiring an acute lower respiratory infection or pneumonia is 1.5-4 times greater among infants who are not breast fed.[4] [18] [22-27] In our study the risk of admission for pneumonia was 17 times greater among infants who were not being breast fed. Even for children who received both maternal and formula milk, the risk was about four times greater than that for children who received breast milk alone. This marked dose-response effect, along with the biological plausi-

- Pneumonia is the leading cause of death in children under 5 years old across the world

- In Brazil infants who were not breast fed were 17 times more likely than those receiving breast milk alone to be admitted for pneumonia

- The relative risk of admission was 61 for children under 3 months of age, decreasing to 10 thereafter

- Supplementation with solids was associated with a relative risk of 13.4 for all infants

- Mothers must be encouraged to breast feed very young infants and be advised of the right time to introduce supplementary foods

Table 4 Odds ratios for developing pneumonia according to type of food given stratified for age

	Cases (n=152)	Controls (n=2391)	Odds ratio (95% CI) Crude	Odds ratio (95% CI) Adjusted*
Age 1-2.9 months				
Type of milk consumed:				
Breast milk alone	5	392	1.0	1.0
Breast and formula milk	7	169	3.2 (1.0 to 10.4)	2.9 (0.8 to 10.5)
Other fluids alone (completely weaned)	35	88	31.2 (11.9 to 81.9)	61.1 (19.0 to 195.5)
P value			<0.001	<0.001
Age 3-5.9 months				
Type of milk consumed:				
Breast milk alone	3	212	1.0	1.0
Breast and formula milk	11	164	4.7 (1.3 to 17.2)	3.4 (0.9 to 13.5)
Other fluids alone (completely weaned)	48	268	12.5 (3.8 to 40.8)	10.1 (2.8 to 36.2)
P value			<0.001	<0.001
Age 6-11.9 months				
Type of milk consumed:				
Breast milk alone	1	175	1.0	1.0
Breast and formula milk	5	230	3.8 (0.4 to 32.9)	3.7 (0.4 to 33.8)
Other fluids alone (completely weaned)	37	693	9.3 (1.3 to 68.6)	9.2 (1.2 to 69.7)
P value			<0.001	<0.01

*For sex, social class, family income, and maternal schooling, age, parity, and weight gained during pregnancy. In addition, each feeding variable was controlled for other two.

Table 5 Simulation to assess effect of misclassification on odds ratios for being admitted for pneumonia for all children

Type of milk consumed	Cases Original (n=152)	Cases Adjusted (n=152)	Controls (n=2391)	Odds ratio Original	Odds ratio Adjusted*
Breast milk alone	9	10.6	779	1.0	1.0
Breast and formula milk	23	43.2	563	3.5	5.6
Other fluids alone (completely weaned)	120	98.2	1049	9.9	6.9

*For sex, social class, family income, and maternal schooling, age, parity, and weight gained during pregnancy.

bility of a link between breast feeding and pneumonia, is strongly supportive of a causal association.[4 18 22]

A Peruvian study investigated whether the protection of breast feeding against respiratory infections changed with age,[24] but it was controlled for few confounding factors. In Brazil the interaction observed was not significant.[22] Further research from Brazil,[23] Argentina,[25] India,[26] and China[27] did not report interactions between age and breast feeding. In our study the protective effect of breast milk was markedly stronger among young infants than at later ages. This finding is biologically plausible since the immature immune system of young infants is likely to render as even more important the protection afforded by breast milk.[3]

Conclusions

The relative risks of pneumonia associated with the introduction of supplementary foods also varied markedly with age. To our knowledge, this interaction had not been previously described in the literature.

This study shows that breast feeding protects infants against pneumonia and that this proctection varies considerably according to infant age. These findings reinforce the need for targeting breastfeeding promotion efforts at the mothers of very young infants and for recommending the timely introduction of supplementary foods.

We particularly thank Alexander M Walker, Department of Epidemiology, Harvard School of Public Health, and Saul S Morris, Department of Epidemiology and Population Health, London School of Hygiene and Tropical Medicine for their critical reading of the manuscript and their generous comments. We thank the three independent referees who diagnosed pneumonia from hospital records: Drs Elaine P Albernaz, Luciani M Oliveira, and Ricardo Halpern.

Contributors: All authors participated in the study proposal. JAC collected and analysed the data and wrote the paper. CGV helped in the data analysis and in editing the paper. FCB, ISS, and JAF discussed main ideas and helped to edit the paper. JAC and CGV are guarantors.

Funding: This study was supported by the European Community, World Health Organisation, and Fundação de Amparo a Pesquisa do Rio Grande do Sul (FAPERGS), Brazil.

Competing interests: None declared.

1 Pio A, Leowski J, Dam HG. The magnitude of the problem of acute respiratory infections. In: Douglas RM, Kerby-Eaton E, eds. *Acute respiratory infections in childhood. Proceedings of an international workshop, Sydney, August 1984.* Adelaide: University of Adelaide, 1985:100-3.
2 Schwartz B, Lipman H, Lob-Levyt J, Gove S. *The aetiology of acute lower respiratory infections among young children in developing countries.* Geneva: World Health Organisation, 1994.
3 Jelliffe DB, Jelliffe EP. *Human milk in the modern world.* Oxford: Oxford University Press, 1978:84-96.
4 Victora CG, Kirkwood B, Ashworth A, Black RE, Rogers S, Sazawal S, et al. Potential interventions for the prevention of childhood pneumonia in developing countries: improving nutrition. *Am J Clin Nutr* (in press).

5 Feachem RG, Koblinski MA. Interventions for the control of diarrhoea diseases among young children: promotion of breast-feeding. *Bull World Health Organ* 1984;62:271-91.
6 Victora CG, Barros FC, Halpern R, Menezes AMB, Horta BL, Tomasi E, et al. Longitudinal study of mother and child population in an urban region of southern Brazil, 1993. Methodological aspects and preliminary results. *Revista de Saúde Pública* 1996;30:34-45.
7 Rodrigues L, Kirkwood BR. Case-control design in the study of common diseases: updates on the demise of the rare disease assumption and the choice of sampling scheme for controls. *Int J Epidemiol* 1990;13:87-93.
8 Bronfman M, Lombardi C, Facchini LA, Victora CG, Barros FC, Beria JU, et al. The operation of the concept of social class in epidemiological studies. *Revista de Saúde Pública* 1988;22:253-65.
9 Dean AG, Dean JA, Coulombier D, Brendel KA, Smith DC, Burton AH, et al. *Epi Info, version 6: a word processing, database, and statistics program for epidemiology on microcomputers.* Atlanta, GA: Centers for Disease Control and Prevention, 1994.
10 Smith PG, Day NE. The design of case-control studies: the influence of confounding and interactions effects. *Int J Epidemiol* 1984;3:356-65.
11 Rossner B. Hypothesis testing: categorical data. In: *Fundamentals of biostatistics.* 4th ed. Boston, MA: Duxbury Press, 1995:345-442.
12 César JA, Victora CG, Santos IS, Barros FC, Albernaz EP, Oliveira LM, et al. Hospitalisation due to pneumonia: the influence of socio-economic and pregnancy factors in a cohort of children in southern Brazil. *Revista de Saúde Pública* 1997;31:53-61.
13 Norussis NJ. *Statistical package for social sciences for Windows.* Chicago, IL: SPSS, 1993.
14 *Epidemiological graphics, estimation and testing package–EGRET.* Washington, DC: Statistics and Research Corporation, 1988.
15 Victora CG. Case-control studies in maternal child health. In: Boerma JT, ed. *Measurement of maternal child mortality, morbidity and health care: interdisciplinay approaches.* Liège: International Union for the Scientific Study of Population, 1992: 85-108.
16 Victora CG. Case-control studies of the influence of breastfeeding on child morbidity and mortality: methodological issues. In: Atkinson SA, Hanson LA, Chandra RK, eds. *Breastfeeding, nutrition, infection and infant growth in developed and emerging countries.* St Johns, Newfoundland: ARTS Biomedical Publishers and Distributors, 1990:405-18.
17 Schlesselmann JJ. *Case-control studies.* New York: Oxford University Press, 1982:27-68.
18 Morris SS. *Risk factors for acute lower respiratory tract infections. Results from five recently completed case-control studies.* London: Maternal and Child Epidemiology Unit, London School of Hygiene Tropical Medicine, 1995: 2-12.

19 Victora CG, Huttly SR, Fuchs SC, Olinto MTA. The role of conceptual frameworks in epidemiological analysis: a hierarchical approach. *Int J Epidemiol* 1997;26:224-7.
20 Labbok M, Krasovec K. Toward consistency in breastfeeding definitions. *Studies in Family Planning* 1990;21:226-30.
21 Barros FC, Victora CG, Vaughan JP. Breastfeeding and socioeconomic status in Southern Brazil. *Acta Paediat Scand* 1986;75:558-62.
22 Victora CG, Smith PG, Vaughan JP, Nobre LC, Lombardi C, Teixeira AMB, et al. Evidence for a strong protective effect of breast-feeding against infant death due to infectious diseases in Brazil. *Lancet* 1987;ii:319-22.
23 Victora CG, Fuchs SC, Flores JA, Fonseca W, Kirkwood B. Risk factors for pneumonia among children in a Brazilian metropolitan area. *Pediatrics* 1994;93:977-85.

24 Brown KH, Black RE, Romana GL, Kanashiro HC. Infant-feeding practices and their relationship with diarrhoea and other diseases in Huascar (Lima), Peru. *Pediatrics* 1989;83:31-40.
25 Cerqueiro MC, Murthag P, Halac A, Avila M, Weissembacher M. Epidemiology of acute respiratory tract infection in children. *Rev Infect Dis* 1990;12:1021-8.
26 Elleasted-Sayed J, Coodin FJ, Dilling LA, Haworth JC. Breastfeeding against infections in Indian Infants. *Can Med Assoc J* 1979;120:295-8.
27 Chen Y, Shunzhang Y, Li W. Artificial feeding and hospitalization in the first 18 months of life. *Pediatrics* 1988;81:58-62.

(Accepted 26 February 1999)

Notes for tutors

UNIT 1

If you are running a week-long short course or a series of seminars, make sure you allocate at least half of the first session (and possibly all of it) for setting ground rules and defining aims and objectives. You will find later that this time is well spent.

The objectives of individual group members never overlap completely with one another and one important task for the group is to distil out some *group* objectives that reflect what most people wish to achieve and give appropriate weight to less popular objectives that are valued by one or two members. One or two individuals may need your help to modify their objectives or work out how to meet them outside the group setting.

Groups often set unrealistic objectives. In particular, they may set out to cover an excessive amount of material in the time available. In addition, objectives can (and should) change as the course unfolds. Initially, members may define their objectives in terms of specific cognitive achievements (for example, "Understand likelihood ratios"), but as the group process evolves, other types of objective (notably psychodynamic or affective ones) may become more important to them (for example, "Be able to teach likelihood ratios to a mixed ability group" or "Be able to value the contribution of all members of a multidisciplinary team and not just focus on the mathematics of a calculation"). You should facilitate a process whereby the group can revisit its original objectives at regular intervals throughout the course.

UNIT 2

A session on the philosophical foundations of evidence-based health care and the ideological issues associated with its application in practice can easily get out of hand. A single-discipline group, such as a firm of hospital doctors, may share (and take for granted) a number of common assumptions, whereas a multidisciplinary group will include members who have a very different perspective (and different unspoken assumptions).

For example, health service managers may see evidence-based health care as fundamentally to do with controlling the behaviour of clinicians (and thereby reducing unacceptable variations in both clinical standards and costs of care). Some nurses may see the "hierarchy of evidence" (with metaanalysis of randomised controlled trials defined as the gold standard of evidence) as devaluing qualitative research and experiential learning. Some senior doctors may be dismissive of qualitative research and others may be ignorant of the essential steps for achieving change in an organisation. They may also come from a work environment where what they say is generally taken by other members of the team to be "correct".

All this makes for a potentially emotive and unproductive session. It is essential to ensure that the group defines specific aims for the session and permits differences of opinion. For example, an aim such as "To explore different definitions of evidence-based health care and the perspective of different professional groups" would enable differences of opinion to be tolerated and encourage the members to view the issues from an angle other than their own. In contrast, an aim such as "For us all to agree on what evidence-based health care is" will probably generate more heat than light!

The reprints in this section are not the last word on the philosophy or ideology of evidence-based practice! Encourage the group members to bring along their own choice of papers and, rather than focusing on which paper is "right" or "best", extract the main arguments from each one and classify them into different categories.

UNIT 3

There is absolutely no substitute for "hands-on" computer work in this session. If you have that provided as part of a course, lucky you. If not, the individuals in the group must be sent to the library or spend time on the Internet trying out their search strategies. Informaticist Reinhard Wentz has said that searching electronic databases is like catching butterflies – a delicate process and you very rarely get a perfect "catch" first time. You must create both the time and the intellectual environment for your group members to experience the trial and error of searching.

UNIT 4

Do not assume that everyone in your group knows what a randomised controlled trial is and understands its meaning. You might like to invite someone to go over the principles of random allocation "as if teaching a group of students" so you do not lose the less experienced members of the group at this first hurdle.

This is the first paper in the workbook with an accompanying critical appraisal checklist. Encourage the group to be positive – it's very easy to "pick holes" in other people's research and some criticism can be made of every published paper. But your students should recognise the practicalities of research (recruitment difficulties, resource limitations, and so on) and avoid dismissing a study entirely just because it isn't perfect. A more productive educational session might centre round, "Given the limitations of this study which you have extracted from the paper, how would you now interpret its findings and what use would you make of them?".

UNIT 5

Statistics (or, more accurately, basic mathematics) is another highly emotive subject. Although most units in the workbook are designed for mixed ability and multidisciplinary groups, this unit may work best if the group is stratified by the members' confidence in statistics (groups usually stratify themselves pretty well using informal methods). Those who are entirely comfortable with the concepts will probably cause you few problems but you may have trouble from "middle of the pack" students who complete the basic NNT exercise quickly and wish to gain reassurance that they have correctly grasped more advanced concepts such as odds ratios. Their questions can be very off-putting to the struggling student, who then becomes even more disillusioned.

We recommend, therefore, that this unit is *not* run as a group session but that you make yourself available to assist individuals or pairs if they need it. You may also like to encourage the more able members of the group to work with the less able. Often, all you need to do is prompt them to fix a time to meet outside the group session.

UNIT 6

Unlike randomised controlled trials, cohort studies are not part of the everyday vocabulary of the average clinician! The large numbers of participants in many cohort studies and the lack of an intervention (which is what many clinicians think clinical trials are about) may make this type of study quite daunting to individuals without formal training in epidemiology. Note that the four-part question population-intervention-comparison-outcome for intervention studies becomes population-exposure-control-outcome for comparative cohort studies. Make sure your group does not argue itself into dismissing all cohort studies because the control group is "not exactly comparable" to the exposed group. In non-randomised designs there are always systematic differences between the groups. The student's task is to see what the researchers did about these differences and the extent to which the differences are likely to have influenced the results.

UNIT 7

If students get seriously stuck on this unit it is probably because one or more of them has failed to grasp the idea that a positive test does not mean the presence of disease. In *How to read a paper* (Chapter 7, pages 97–99) this problem is addressed using the example of a jury verdict. Almost everyone knows that a jury can find someone guilty when they committed no crime and find them innocent when they are not. Hence, the "test result" is the jury's verdict while the "gold standard" is whether the criminal knows in his or her heart that they committed the crime! Once students have understood this concept, they should be able to follow the steps involved in a validation study.

The other potential problem in this unit is the likelihood ratio (and receiver operator characteristic or ROC curves). Likelihood ratios and ROC curves are elegant and useful and when this concept "clicks" the student often feels they have made a real breakthrough in grasping the concepts of EBHC. But don't forget that this is one full step beyond the basics and if your group is new to concepts like sensitivity, specificity and predictive value, you are likely to encounter difficulties if you allow a general discussion of likelihood ratios in the same session. You may choose to split the group at this stage – suggesting, for example, that those who have "had enough" go for a teabreak at this point so that they do not become confused. You can offer to cover the more advanced concepts for them at a later stage or, better, invite the more experienced members of the group to explain them to their colleagues on an individual basis.

UNIT 8

If students find this unit on systematic review daunting, it may be because many people believe (wrongly) that it is about complex mathematics. You should make sure that this session begins with an exploration of what systematic review is all about – it's not simply about adding up the results of lots of studies in a particular way. The defining feature of a systematic review is that it has a *methods* section so the reader can make an independent judgement about the appropriateness of the question, the thoroughness of the search, the criteria used to dismiss papers as irrelevant or poor quality, and so on. Students often need encouragement to focus initially on what the reviewer *did* rather than on the "bottom line" of what they said they found.

UNIT 9

A session on qualitative research is likely to be viewed as a welcome relief by some members, a pointless digression by others, and a threat to the foundations of "pure" evidence-based medicine by a substantial minority. Although a discussion about whether qualitative research should "count" in clinical epidemiology may be very useful, your group must decide whether

155

they want to focus on such philosophical issues or tackle the content of the paper and do the checklist! Your task is to help them make this decision and ensure that they meet their objective, not to get drawn into taking sides in the somewhat spurious "qualitative versus quantitative" debate! You will probably need all your facilitation skills in this unit but in our experience, this session can be particularly worthwhile as one or more group members come to grasp the idea of an entirely new paradigm.

UNIT 10

Make sure everyone in the group is clear about the difference between a case control study (in which putative harmful agents are looked for *retrospectively* in patients who have already developed a disease) and a comparative cohort study (in which people exposed to the putative agent are followed up *prospectively* to see what proportion get the disease – as illustrated in Unit 6). Both these designs may be used to assess "harm". Case control studies usually sink or swim on the comparability of cases and controls, so the exploration of potential systematic biases here is crucial. However, as we explained in the notes for Unit 6, no non-randomised trial is entirely free of bias or confounding so the reader needs to exercise judgement!

Model answers for checklists

UNIT 4: RANDOMISED CONTROLLED TRIALS OF THERAPY

1. The trial did address a clearly focused question: "In patients referred to secondary care with newly diagnosed non-ketotic type 2 diabetes, who also have raised blood pressure (BP), will 'tight' control of BP to a target of <150/85 reduce mortality, macrovascular morbidity or microvascular morbidity, compared with 'less tight' control to a target BP of <180/105?".
2. Trial participants were not randomly selected. Rather, all patients from the population (newly diagnosed non-ketotic type 2 diabetics with hypertension referred to secondary care) who met the inclusion criteria were offered the opportunity to participate.
3. Allocation was randomised by means of sealed opaque envelopes.
4. Neither participants nor observers were blinded. Since the intervention included different target BPs for each group, blinding of clinicians would not have been possible, but blind assessment of complications by a different observer would have been theoretically possibly. Participants could have been blinded by the use of placebo tablets.
5. The two groups were treated equally in that there was no difference in the frequency of clinic visits or the assessment protocol.
6. No power calculation is given. The hypertension substudy of UKPDS has been criticised for being underpowered to test its most important hypothesis – that tight vs less tight control of BP in type 2 diabetes produces a significant reduction in all-cause mortality.
7. Ninety-six percent of participants were accounted for at the end of the study (page 67). Results were analysed on an intention-to-treat basis (i.e. in the groups to which they were randomised).
8. The predefined primary endpoints are listed at the top of page 67. Examples of the main results, shown graphically in Figure 4, were:

End point (or outcome)	Relative risk (95% CI)	Relative risk reduction (RRR = 1-RR)	Absolute risk reduction (= CER-EER)	NNT (=1/ARR)
All diabetes-related outcomes	0.76 (0.62–0.92)	0.24	9.4% (i.e. 0.094)	11
All-cause mortality	0.82 (0.63–1.08)	0.18	3.6% (i.e. 0.036)	28
MI	0.79 (0.59–1.07)	0.21	3.6% (i.e. 0.036)	28

9. The estimates of treatment effect are, for many outcomes, imprecise, as shown by the wide confidence intervals in Figure 4. Where these intervals overlap the line of no effect (relative risk of 1.0), we cannot be sure whether this is due to a type 2(β) error or whether there is genuinely no difference in efficacy between the treatment regimens.
10. The study participants were all newly diagnosed non-ketotic diabetic patients referred to UK secondary care and selected on the basis of a long list of inclusion and exclusion criteria (page 65). Notable exclusions were those with long established diabetes, those managed exclusively in primary care, those over 65, and those whose glycaemia was adequately controlled on diet alone.

UNIT 5: THE FIRST EVER RANDOMISED CONTROLLED TRIAL

The event rate for death in the experimental group (EER)
EER = a/a+b = 4/55 = 0.07

The event rate for death in the control group (CER)
CER = c/c+d = 14/52 = 0.27

The absolute risk reduction (ARR) for the outcome death
ARR = CER − EER = 0.27 − 0.07 = 0.20 = 20%

The relative risk reduction (RRR) for the outcome death
RRR = (CER − EER) / CER
= (0.27 − 0.07)/0.27 = 0.2/0.27 + 0.74 = 74%

The number needed to treat (NNT) to prevent one death
NNT = 1/ARR = 1/0.20 = 5
Five patients must receive streptomycin to prevent one additional death.

The chance (risk) of death in the experimental and control groups respectively
Risk of death is the same as the event rate, i.e. 0.07 in the experimental group and 0.27 in the control group.

The odds of death in the experimental and control groups respectively
Odds of death   = number of patients dying/number of patients not dying
                 = a/b = 4/51 = 0.078 in the experimental group
                 = c/d = 14/38 = 0.37 in the control group

The relative risk (risk ratio) for death in the experimental group compared with the control group
Risk ratio   = risk in experimental group/risk in control group
              = 0.07/0.27
              = 0.26

The relative odds (odds ratio) for death in the experimental group compared with the control group
Odds ratio   = odds in experimental group/odds in control group
             = 0.07/0.37
             = 0.21

The number needed to harm (NNH) for the outcome VIIIth nerve damage

	VIIIth nerve damage		Total
	Yes	No	
Experimental (streptomycin) group	36 a	b 19	55
Control group (bed rest alone)	0 c	d 52	52

CER for VIIIth nerve damage = 0
EER for VIIIth nerve damage = 36/55 = 0.65
NNH = 1/(CER − EER) = 1/(0 − 0.65) = −1/0.65 = −1.5
i.e. one person develops deafness for every 1.5 people treated (or two develop deafness for every three treated). The NNH is a negative number because the experimental group do worse than the controls for this outcome.

The 95% confidence interval for the NNT is 2.98–17.31, a fairly wide limit which reflects the small sample size.

UNIT 6: COHORT STUDIES

1. The trial did address a clearly focused question: "In women who were ever prescribed the combined oral contraceptive pill by their GP, compared to those who have never taken this drug, what is the risk of death over the subsequent 25 years?"
2. The study was prospective. Note that GPs were asked to record contraceptive use *prospectively* every six months.

3. The groups were registered with the same GPs. Major potentially confounding variables – age, social class, parity and cigarette smoking at recruitment – were assessed at the outset and controlled for in the subsequent analysis. That said, a legitimate question might be: "were women who took the pill systematically different in sexual activity (and hence disease risk) from those who did not?" The study does not control for sexual activity. A book is cited (reference 1) that may give important data on this question.

4. Follow-up was 75% because 25% of the original 1968 cohort were lost to long-term follow-up before it was "flagged" in 1976–7. Some (we are not told what proportion) of these 25% of participants were lost because their GP withdrew from the study, others presumably withdrew for their own reasons. We are told that women who withdrew had similar mortality patterns to those who remained in follow-up, but we are not given the data from which this statement is derived. All participants who *were* followed up were analysed on an intention-to-treat basis.

5. Results are given as relative risk with 95% confidence intervals. Outcomes were overall and cause-specific mortality, both in total and broken down by years since first exposure. Over 25 years, the relative risk of all-cause mortality from oral contraceptive use compared to "never used" was 1.0, i.e. there was no excess long-term harm associated with the pill, while the relative risk of death from "all circulatory diseases" (for example, the pulmonary embolus that your patient is concerned about) was 1.7 (95% CI 1.2–2.4) (Table 1, page 95). Within the first 10 years, however, relative risks fo the different conditions were higher (Table 2).

6. With 46,000 patients, it is not surprising that the data on all-cause mortality are very precise. For all-cause mortality at 25 years, 95% confidence intervals were 0.9–1.1. However, data on less common cause-specific mortality are less precise, for example, relative risk of death from liver cancer was 5.0, with a 95% confidence interval of 0.6–43.2! The 95% confidence intervals for the relative risk of "other circulatory diseases" are 0.8–2.5, i.e. there is a high chance that the slight excess mortality observed in this study arose by chance.

7. This depends on your circumstances. It might be helpful to note that this paper focuses on *long-term mortality*. It gives no data on short-term, non-fatal outcomes such as venous thrombosis or minor pulmonary embolism. Second, the patient in the scenario given is probably from a non-white or mixed ethnicity, whereas the participants in the study were almost all white (page 92). Third, the dose of contraceptive that this patient plans to take will be lower than that taken by pill users in the 1960s and 1970s. Fourth, the women in the study were "living as married", this patient may or may not be in a stable relationship. Finally, patterns of disease have changed considerably since the 1970s. In particular, HIV-related illness accounts for a substantial proportion of deaths in young women. Hence, the use of barrier contraceptive methods (as well as, or instead of, taking the pill) may have a greater impact on outcome in this patient than it did in the study participants.

UNIT 7: DIAGNOSTIC OR SCREENING TESTS

1. The paper implies, but does not state explicitly, that the investigator who administered the "gold standard" diagnostic alcohol use interview was blind to the results of the self-administered screening questionnaire and that those who calculated the score from the latter were blind to the result of the diagnostic interview.

2. The test was evaluated in a sample of primary care patients who were attending their GP for an unrelated condition on the day of interview. In this respect, the participants are similar to the patient in the case history.

3. The low prevalence of people with alcohol problems in the population (most interviewees scored negative on both tests and there was no attempt, for example, to oversample from patients with risk factors for alcohol excess) casts some doubt on its usefulness in the specific subgroup of patients whom we *suspect* are misusing alcohol. Ideally, a new test should be compared with the gold standard in patients in whom there is a high degree of diagnostic uncertainty before the test result is known, especially in patients with mild forms of the disease and commonly confused conditions. A power calculation is not included in the paper.

4. Both tests were used on all participants.

5. The 10-item questionnaire, using a cut-off score of 5, had a sensitivity of 84%, a specificity of 90%, and a positive predictive value of 60%. For the five-item questionnaire these figures were 79%, 95%, and 73% respectively. The question of whether these values are "good enough" has no hard and fast answer. In general, a screening test should be highly sensitive (but not necessarily specific) since false-positive cases can be excluded by a more definitive test. The figures for sensitivity tell us that a 10-item questionnaire will miss one case in six and the five-item questionnaire one case in five of serious alcohol problems. The figures for positive predictive value tell us that (in this population) a person who scores "positive" on the 10-item questionnaire has a 60% chance and someone who scores positive on the five-item questionnaire has a 73% chance of having a serious alcohol problem.

6. According to an international study cited in the paper, 6% of primary care attenders worldwide have a serious alcohol problem. The prevalence in any particular practice may vary from this and if it does, the features of the test (the positive and negative predictive values) will change. (You can test this out for yourself by replacing the starting prevalence figures [73, 409] in the total boxes at the base of the "condition present" and "condition absent" columns below.)

7. The study population here had a prevalence of 16% (73/482). Using these figures, there was a good chance that if the patient tested negative, they did *not* have the disease (97% – the negtive predictive value = 368/380). If your population has a *lower* prevalence than this (e.g. 6%, like the overall population), then the negative predictive value is likely to be even higher and the test more useful to you for ruling out non-alcoholics. On the other hand, with 16% prevalence, this test has a low positive predictive value (60% [61/102] meaning that there is a 40% chance that a positive result occurs in someone *without* the condition). If your prevalence is lower, then the positive predictive value will fall further, making a positive test result not very useful at all (no better than tossing a coin, for example).

8. In the case history described in Unit 7, a negative result would be reassuring, as you may feel that the patient does not need a long face-to-face interview (or even a confrontation) to address his alleged alcohol problem. A positive result should probably change your management by at least indicating a more definitive test. Whether your patients would be willing to be treated is a difficult question that is important to address (but is not addressed by this paper). There may be other papers in the research literature which may help to estimate how likely it is that patients detected by primary care screening would accept (and respond to) treatment for alcohol misuse.

9. The paper suggests that the test is simple, cheap, and acceptable but this would need to be tested in your own practice, preferably by a formal feasibility study.

Note: The authors did not supply raw data in their paper, but if you are curious and wish to see how the 2×2 matrix would look, the following figures are consistent with the results in the paper for the full 10-item questionnaire. (We derived these figures from the data supplied in the paper.)

		Target disorder		Totals
		Present	Absent	
Diagnostic test result	Positive	61	41	102
	Negative	12	368	380
	Totals	73	409	482

Sensitivity = 61/73 = 84%
Specificity = 368/409 = 90%
Prevalence in the study = 73/482 = 15%
Positive predictive value (in the study) = 61/102 = 60%
Negative predictive value (in the study) = 368/380 = 97%
Likelihood ratio of a positive test = sensitivity/1-specificity = 8.34

UNIT 8: SYSTEMATIC REVIEWS

1. Yes. "In patients with asthma sensitive to house dust mite, what is the impact of physical and chemical methods to control mites on the symptoms of asthma or allergy and/or on peak expiratory flow rate?"

2. Yes. Of 229 studies identified from a literature search, all but 18 were excluded as irrelevant or of poor quality. An additional four studies were known to one of the authors. All these studies were described as randomised; 11 were double blind. However, only one of the papers contained sufficient information to confirm that randomisation was adequately concealed. All the studies addressed the research question above. All contained relatively small numbers of participants.

3. It is unlikely that important relevant studies were missed. A sensitive search strategy was used on several databases. References of references in all 233 studies were pursued, but no additional studies were identified.

4. Validity of studies was assessed by a reproducible method (available on the web version of the paper). It is unclear whether more than one assessor graded the primary studies independently.

5. Broadly, the results were similar from study to study. However, there appeared to be some heterogeneity of effect size between chemical methods and physical methods, with the former producing neutral or negative effects and the latter producing more positive effects on symptoms

(Figure 2). Given the small numbers in some of the subgroups, there may be a genuine heterogeneity in the effect of these different methods and if there is, it would not be valid to express the results of this metaanalysis as a single "grand mean".

6. The point estimate of overall effect of size is close to zero (but see point 5 above).
7. The confidence intervals on the aggregated data are narrow.
8. All the participants in this study had documented house dust mite allergy. Compliance with the regimen was only evaluated in one study and the lack of effect of some measures may have been partly explained by lack of compliance. Hence, highly motivated patients who comply strictly with the regimen may *theoretically* experience greater benefit but this hypothesis would need to be tested in a separate trial.
9. Outcomes included both symptoms (asthma and allergy) and peak expiratory flow rate. Different trials used different outcomes. There may be additional outcomes (for example, days lost from school or work) that were not measured in some or all studies.

UNIT 9: QUALITATIVE RESEARCH

1. Yes. The aim was to explore the reasons why patients with a cardiac event did or did not take appropriate action.
2. Yes. The authors sought to explain the variation in response to a cardiac event and identify potentially modifiable factors.
3. Yes. The sample comprised all patients admitted to a district general hospital who had survived a cardiac event.
4. It may have been useful to study patients with non-cardiac causes for their chest pain and those with cardiac events (if any) who were not admitted to hospital.
5. Yes. Subjects all had confirmed acute myocardial infarction.
6. No. Little detail is given on the researchers' background. The researchers do not comment on how their background or perspective may have influenced the findings.
7. Yes. Data sources were semistructured interviews with patients and relatives or bystanders. These were appropriate. Focus groups would have been another useful method that may have provided additional data.
8. Partly. The length of the interviews, the questions asked, and themes covered were all given. Additional detail on the setting and format of the interview, the reasons given by the researchers for seeking the information, and the manner in which questions were posed could have been supplied. Patients and relatives or bystanders were both interviewed. The interviews were audiotaped so were independently verifiable. Observations were not taken at different times. The approach was highly standardised, with patients being interviewed on the third or fourth day post event: informants were all interviewed in a hospital setting on the same afternoon, before they saw the patient. This was clearly done for practical reasons but more variety in the context and timing of the interview might have produced additional data.
9. Yes. "The data were analysed using the constant comparative method to cover identified and emerging themes" – a reference to this standard method is given and an accompanying commentary explains its theoretical basis. Agreement was reached in all but three cases – we are not told how these were resolved. It was not clear how the authors dealt with negative or discrepant results.
10. The results show that patients can be classified as "non-delayers", "delayers", and "extended delayers" and each of these categories displays different perceptions and behaviours. For example, extended delayers were characterised by low perception of own risk for a cardiac event, atypical (non-dramatic) symptoms, evolving symptoms, multiple attempts at self-treatment, and inappropriate advice given by lay advisers and health professionals. The results are coherent and do address the research question.
11. Yes; they are consistent with the data. All information is available for independent assessment.
12. Yes.
13. Public perceptions of the nature of a heart attack and its associated symptoms need to be changed. In particular, the stereotype of a sudden, dramatic and all-or-nothing event must change to reflect the reality of less dramatic, evolving symptoms in many cases.
14. Depends.
15. Yes, if your practice is the acute management of patients with chest symptoms in the UK.

UNIT 10: CASE CONTROL STUDIES

1. Yes. "In infants born in Petolas, Brazil and living in urban areas, is exclusive breast feeding associated with a reduced incidence of pneumonia between the ages of one and twelve months, compared to infants given fluid supplements, those on mixed (formula plus breast) feeding, and those given solid supplements?"

2. Fairly uncommon. The incidence of pneumonia in the postneonatal period in these infants was 2.9%.

3. The study was population based.

4. Controls were slightly older, of slightly higher social class, and their mothers had more education but fewer children. All these factors were shown in the study to be independently associated with protection against pneumonia. After adjustment for these variables (far right column, Tables 3 and 4), the odds ratios for development of pneumonia in each subcategory are reduced but still highly significant.

5. The study was not matched at the individual level. Rather, it was a *nested* case control study in which the small number of cases (infants with pneumonia) were compared with the pooled data on all infants in the sample from the cohort study.

6. Outcome was hospital admission with pneumonia independently diagnosed from records by two paediatricians. The adjusted odds ratio for the effect of exposure to breast plus formula milk compared to breast milk alone was 3.8 across all age groups studied. Fluid supplementation (e.g. with water or herb tea) had an adjusted odds ratio of 1.3 compared with no supplementation and solid supplements an adjusted odds ratio of 8.5 compared with no solids.

7. The 95% confidence intervals for the three figures given above are 1.7–8.9, 0.3–4.9 and 4.7–15.4.

8. Dr Sawar's population is rural rather than urban, Indian rather than Brazilian, and probably of lower socioeconomic status and educational level. Although there is a highly plausible pathological explanation for a "dose response" effect of supplementary feeding in any population of infants, there are major differences between the study population and the one this doctor cares for. He should seek additional evidence from the clinical literature but, if he does not find it, he must make a personal judgement about the generalisability of these findings to his own practice.

Index

absolute risk reduction (ARR) 81, 83, 158
abstracts, structured 21, 55–6
accuracy 97, 99
adherence, to medication 142
"adj" operator 44
Agency for Health Care Policy and Research, clinical
    guidelines 52–3, 56
AIDSLINE 46
"AIM journals" option 44
aims 1–2
Alcohol Use Disorders Identification Test 97, 98,
    101–9, 159–60
alcohol use, harmful, screening for 98, 101–9,
    159–60
Allied and Alternative Medicine 46
American College of Physicians (ACP) Journal Club 19,
    22, 53
American Hospital Association 54
American Medical Association Journals database 46
amoxycillin, in non-suppurative otitis media 122
"and" operator 41
anecdotes, personal 142
anticoagulation, in atrial fibrillation 18, 19, 20–1
antidepressants 121–2
appraisal, critical *see* critical appraisal
articles
    critical appraisal *see* critical appraisal
    individual study 4–5
    quality filters 45–6, 48, 54
    searching for specific 40–2
    structured abstracts 21, 55–6
ASSIA database 46
asthma
    house dust mite control measures 111–12, 114–19,
        160–1
    qualitative research 141–2
atrial fibrillation, anticoagulation in 18, 19, 20–1
audit 28

Bandolier 53
best available external clinical evidence 14
Best Evidence Database on CD ROM 53
bias
    "criteria" 31
    location 127
    publication 120, 127
Biomednet 54
blinding 30
blood pressure control, in diabetes 59, 60, 62–72
boolean operators 41, 44

Bradford Hill, Sir Austin 80
brainstorming 38
breast feeding, impact on pneumonia in infants
    145–6, 148–52, 162
British Medical Association (BMA) 23
    library 55
British Medical Journal 42, 56

Canadian Guide to Clinical Preventive Health Care
    53
Cancer-CD database 46
cardiac events, patients' actions during 131, 132,
    135–9, 161
case control studies 85, 145–51
    critical appraisal 146–7, 162
    nested 162
    notes for tutors 156
    population based 147, 148
    set article 145, 148–52
CD-ROM subscriptions 23
chest pain, patients' actions during 132, 135–9, 161
cholesterol lowering therapy 123
CINAHL database 46
clinical effectiveness
    evaluating 23
    finding information on 51–7
clinical experience 141
clinical expertise
    importance 33
    individual, definition 14
clinical guidelines 52–3, 56
clinical practice
    implementing change 56
    limits of objectivity 33
    narrative based 33–5
    relation to study designs 31
clinical significance 83–4
clinicians
    computer skills 23–4
    learning evidence based medicine 22
    senior *see* senior clinicians
Cochrane, Archie 125
Cochrane Collaboration 125–6
Cochrane Database of Systematic Reviews 19, 124–5
Cochrane Library 46, 52
coding data 139–40
cohort studies 89–96
    comparative 89, 156
    critical appraisal 90, 158–9
    notes for tutors 154–5

communication, between health workers 23
computers
    cost implications 23
    for searching databases 18
    skills 23–4, 154
confidence intervals 79, 81–2, 84
    in meta-analyses 126
constant comparative method 136, 139–40, 161
consumers 22
content, learning 3
continuity of care 23
contraceptive advice 89–91, 158–9
control event rate (CER) 80–1, 85, 158
coronary artery bypass surgery 123–4
coronary heart disease, mortality 123
costs
    cutting 15
    evidence based medicine 23
critical appraisal 19–21
    clinical guidelines 56
    collections 54
    questions 20
cross sectional studies, delayed type 30
Current Contents Search 46
Current Research in Britain 46

data
    analysis, subjectivity in 122
    coding 139–40
    individual patient, for meta-analyses 123–4, 127
    presentation, clear 21
    reporting, subjectivity in 122
    unpublished, in meta-analyses 120–2
databases, electronic 18–19, 46–7, 52–5 see also
        Medline database
    access to 55
    disadvantages 23–4
    searching see searching the literature
    types available 19
Department of Health 46, 52
depression, antidepressants in 121–2
DHData (formerly DHSS-Data) 46
Diabetes Control and Complications Trial (DCCT)
        83–4
diabetes mellitus 60
    blood pressure control 59, 60, 62–72
diagnosis, narrative based 34–5
diagnostic tests 15, 97–109
    calculations 99
    derivation of features 99
    notes for tutors 155
    objective analysis 35
    validation study
        2x2 table 98, 160
        critical appraisal 100, 159–60
dissemination of evidence 51–7
doctors see clinicians
Drug and Therapeutics Bulletin 53

Effective Health Care Bulletin 53
Effectiveness Matters 53
effect size, point estimate of 82

elderly, hypertension in 123
electronic databases see databases, electronic
Embase 47
event rate
    control (CER) 80–1, 85, 158
    experimental (EER) 81, 85, 158
    patient expected (PEER) 86
evidence
    appraising see critical appraisal
    availability 52–5
    best available external clinical 14
    dissemination 51–7
    gaps 23
    hierarchy 153
    implementing 21, 56
    internal vs external validity 30–1
    medicine based 30–1
    quality filters 45–6, 48, 54
    searching for see searching the literature
    strategies for finding and filtering 55
evidence based health care (EBHC)
    definition 11
    differences of opinion 153
    notes for tutors 153–4
    principles and practice 11–35
evidence based medicine 14–16, 17–24
    advantages 22–3
    criticisms 14
    definitions 14, 17–18, 30
    disadvantages 23–4
    effectiveness 22
    evolution 15
    four steps 18–21
    medicine based evidence for 30–1
    misunderstandings about 14–15
    in practice see evidence based practice
Evidence Based Medicine (journal) 53
evidence based practice
    applied to individual patient 27–8
    definition 14
    evaluating one's own performance 26–8
    requirements for 18–22
    surveys 26–7
    workshops for teaching 8–9
evidence based quality filters (EBQF) 45–6, 48
examinations, individual study for 4
experiential text 35
experimental event rate (EER) 81, 85, 158
expertise, clinical, see clinical expertise
experts, consulting 4
"explode" command 45

feedback, giving 4
Fibrinolytic Therapy Trialists' Collaborative Group
        123

General Medical Council 6–7
general practice
    access to databases 55
    evidence based practice 26, 27
Grateful Med 54–5
grounded theory 139–40

groups
 aims 1–2
 ground rules 3
 learning 2–4
  basics 3–4
  set article 2, 6–9
  structure 3–4
 notes for tutors 153
 rules for giving feedback 4
Gruppo Italiano per lo Studio della Streptochinasi nell'Infarto Miocardico 126
Guide to Clinical Preventive Services, 2nd edition 53
guidelines, clinical 52–3, 56

harm, assessing 156
Harvard Medical School, new pathway programme 6, 8
health service managers 153
HealthSTAR database 54
heart attack see myocardial infarction
HELMIS 47
help seeking behaviour 135–9
house dust mite control measures 111–12, 114–19, 160–1
hypertension
 in diabetes 59, 60, 62–72
 in elderly 123

illness behaviour 135–9
"illness scripts" 34–5
implementation of evidence 21, 56
individual study 4–5
 aims and objectives 1, 2
infants
 formula milks 146
 impact of breast feeding on pneumonia 145–6, 148–52, 162
information professionals 55
instrumental text 35
internet Grateful Med 54–5
in vivo codes 139–40

Journal of the American Medical Association (JAMA) 42, 46
 series of user's guides 20
journal clubs 22
journals
 access to information not in 54
 articles see articles
 editors 56
 medical see medical journals
 nursing 44

Knowledge Finder searching software 19

language, Medline articles 44
learning
 content 3
 deep 2–3
 objectives 1, 2, 153
 problem based, small group 6–9
 process 3
 superficial 2

librarians 55
libraries 55
 outreach services 55
likelihood ratio 97, 98, 155, 160
"limit set" option 43–4, 45
literature, research 37–58
 generating clinical questions 37–9
 searching see searching the literature

McMaster University Medical School, Canada 6, 8, 18
 Health Information Research Unit 56
mean 82
medical informatics 55
medical journals
 data presentation 21
 mainstream ("AIM") 44
medical students
 learning evidence based medicine 22
 problem based learning 6–7
medical subject headings (MESH) 40, 42
 "explode" command 45
medication
 adherence to 142
 attitudes to 142
medicine, general, evidence based practice 26
Medline database 19, 23, 40–50
 access to 54–5
 alternative sources of information 46–7
 combining two/more broad searches 42–3
 evidence based quality filters 45–6, 48
 "explode" command 45
 field suffix or textword searches 40–2
 limitations 54–5
 maximally sensitive search strings 49–50
 "permuted index" option 45
 refining the search 44
 search gives no/too few articles 45
 using subheadings and/or "limit set" options 43–4, 45
MeReC Bulletin 54
MESH see medical subject headings
meta-analyses 31, 111–29 see also systematic reviews
 clinical application of results 126
 Cochrane Collaboration 125
 distrust of results 126
 notes for tutors 155
 outlook 127
 subjectivity in data analysis and reporting 122
 summary statistics vs individual patient data 123–4
 unpublished data 120–2
 unresolved issues 120–6
 value of "failed" 124–5
Midwives Information and Resource Service 56
myocardial infarction
 patients' actions during 131, 132, 135–9, 161
 thrombolysis after 123, 126

narrative based medicine 33–5
narrative text 35
National Information Center on Health Services Research and Health Care Technology (US) 55

National Library of Medicine (US) 54–5
National Network of Libraries of Medicine (US) 55
negative predictive value 99, 160
New England Journal of Medicine 126
NHS Economic Evaluation Database 54
NNT *see* number needed to treat
"not" operator 44
number needed to harm (NNH) 79, 81, 158
number needed to treat (NNT) 79, 83–4, 85
   calculation 81, 85, 158
   for specific patients 84
   translating odds ratio to 86, 87
nurses 153
nursing journals 44

objectives, learning 1, 2, 153
objectivity, limits to, in clinical method 33
odds 81, 158
odds ratio (OR) 79, 85–7
   calculation 81, 158
   in case control studies 147, 162
   disadvantages 86–7
   origins 85–6
   translation to number needed to treat 86, 87
oral contraceptive pill 89–91, 92–6, 158–9
"or" operator 41
otitis media, amoxycillin, in non-suppurative 122
outcomes
   in meta-analyses 124
   subjective choice of 122
outreach library services 55
Ovid Technologies software 40, 42
Oxford Health Libraries' training programme 55
Oxford PRISE project 55

papers *see* articles
patient expected event rates (PEERs) 86
patients
   actions during cardiac events 131, 132, 135–9, 161
   attitudes to medication 142
   generalising evidence to individual 30–1
   priorities for individual 27–8
perceptual text 35
"permuted index" option 45
physical text 35
pneumonia, in infants, impact of breast feeding 145–6, 148–52, 162
point estimate of effect size 82
Population–Exposure–Outcome (PEO) 37–8, 90, 155
Population–Intervention–Comparison–Outcome (PICO) 37–8
positive predictive value 99, 159, 160
post-test likelihood of a negative test 97, 99
post-test likelihood of a positive test 97, 99
predictive value
   negative 99, 160
   positive 99, 159, 160
pre-randomisation 30
pre-test likelihood 97
prevalence, in study population 97, 99, 160
probability 81

problem based, small group learning 6–9
process, learning 3
prognosis 15, 89
psychiatry, evidence based practice 26
Psychlit 47
publication bias 120, 127
PubMed 54–5
purchasers 22

qualitative research 131–43
   assessing 142
   critical appraisal 132–3, 161
   evidence based medicine and 141–3
   interaction and relativism 142
   interpretation 141
   naturalism 141
   notes for tutors 155–6
   process 141–2
   set articles 131, 135–42
quasi-experimental methods 31
questions
   clinical
      answerable from literature 37–8
      generating 18, 37–9
      Medline search strategies 42–3
   critical appraisal 20

randomised controlled trials 15, 31, 59–78
   compared to non-randomised trials 59, 73–8
   critical appraisal 61, 157
   first ever 80–1, 158
   notes for tutors 154
   set article 59, 62–72
receiver operator characteristic (ROC) curves 155
relative odds *see* odds ratio
relative risk (RR) 79, 85
   calculation 81, 158
   in case control studies 147
   reduction (RRR) 83
      calculation 81, 158
      vs odds ratio 85, 86
"restrict to focus" 42
risk 81, 158
   avoidance, by researchers 31
   relative *see* relative risk
risk ratio 79, 81
role play 8
Royal College of General Practitioners' oral contraceptive study 89, 92–6
Russell, Bertrand 40

sample size 82
Science Citation Index 47
Scientific American on CD-ROM 19
screening tests 97–109
   calculations 99
   derivation of features 99
   hazardous alcohol use 98, 101–9
   notes for tutors 155
   validation study
      2x2 table 98, 160
      critical appraisal 100, 159–60

searching the literature 18–19
  Medline database *see* Medline database
  notes for tutors 154
  problems in 23–4
  strategies 55
selective serotonin uptake inhibitors 121–2
senior clinicians
  attitudes of 24, 153
  support from 22
sensitivity 97, 99, 159
  calculation 99, 160
SHARE 47
Silver Platter Information software (WinSPIRS) 40, 42
specificity 97, 99
  calculation 99, 160
standard deviation 82
standard error 82
statistics 79–87
  notes for tutors 154
  set articles 79, 83–7
  worked example 80–1, 158
streptomycin, in tuberculosis 80–1, 158
stroke, acute ischaemic 124–5
study designs, relation to clinical practice 31
studying alone *see* individual study
subgroup analyses 31, 123–4
subheadings, Medline 43–4, 45
subjectivity, in data analysis and reporting 122
summary statistics, in meta-analyses 123–4
systematic reviews 15, 52, 111–27 *see also* meta-analyses
  collections 54
  critical appraisal 113, 160–1
  methods section 111, 155
  notes for tutors 155
  odds ratios 85–7

textbooks, reference 4
therapy 15
  clinically useful measures of effects 83–4
  critical appraisal of articles on 20
  narratives 35
  trials *see* randomised controlled trials
thrombolysis
  in acute ischaemic stroke 124–5
  in acute myocardial infarction 123, 126
time, needed for evidence based medicine 23
time out/time in markers 3
timetables, for individual study 4
Toxline 47
treatment *see* therapy
tuberculosis, streptomycin in 80–1, 158
tutors, notes for 153–6

UNICORN 47
uniformity of care 23
United Kingdom
  Consortium on Teaching Evidence-Based Medicine 8–9
  undergraduate medical education 6–7
  workshops for teaching evidence based practice 8–9
United Kingdom Prospective Diabetes Study (UKPDS) Group 59, 60, 62–72
  critical appraisal 61, 157
University College London (UCL) Medical School, London 8–9

validity, internal vs external 30–1

warfarin, in atrial fibrillation 18, 19, 20–1
workshops, for teaching evidence based practice 8–9, 20

York Centre for Reviews and Dissemination 23